HEALING MATTERS

Celebrating Women's Innate Healing Nature

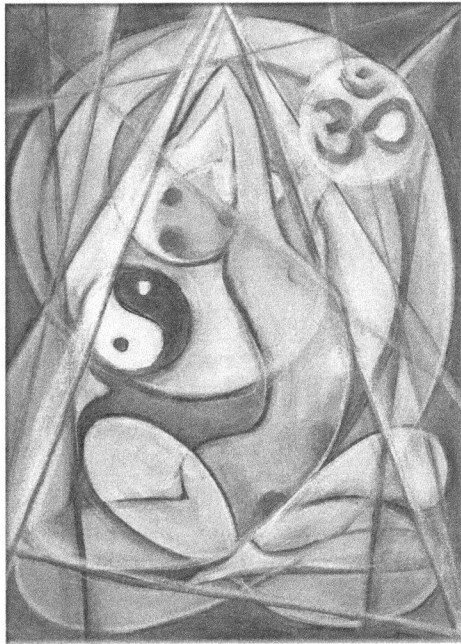

PAMELA SKY JEANNE, ND

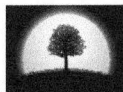

SKY VIEW
PRESS

Healing Matters:
Celebrating Women's Innate Healing Nature

Pamela Sky Jeanne, ND

ISBN: 978-1-936214-81-5
Library of Congress Control Number: 2012936090

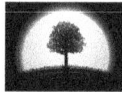

SKY VIEW
P R E S S

Published by Sky View Press, A Wyatt-MacKenzie Imprint
www.WyattMacKenzie.com

Dedicated to

My life partner – Sarah

and

Every woman who cares for others
Past...
      Present...
           Future...

"The world cannot do without women...

The future lies with us."

~Joan Collins Actor, Author, Columnist

TABLE OF CONTENTS

Acknowledgments

I am so grateful for living during this time of ease for publishing one's work. The idea of writing came slowly over the last few years and my first inspiration came from Karen Waters who held a lovely class called "Women Writing for (a)Change" in Portland. My decision to join the class allowed me to dip my toe into this new adventure of actually writing a book! It was a fabulously supportive environment and I am so grateful to Karen and all the women in her classes. I began to write...

Jessica Glenn and Eva Silva teamed up to help me begin sorting through my material and creating my first chapters. They were inspirational women who gave me a great start. Thank you.

My thanks to Charlotte Rains Dixon who assisted in further writing and organizing. I am so grateful to have had her talent in continuing to shape this work.

My greatest thanks goes to Susan Adams. With each editing she completed, my ideas became refined and clearer. Her talent and attention to details along with her kind and poignant questions has made this work better than I could imagine. I am in deep gratitude for her graciousness in helping me with this important work. I have felt her support and encouragement along the way.

I am grateful for the NCNM (National College of Natural Medicine) community for being the great resource and education in healing. You have taught me and continue to teach me and many others. Special thanks to David J. Schleich, PhD, the college president, for his initial encouragement and words. In releasing this work I encourage all students of healing arts: Allopathic, Naturopathic, Ayurvedic, Traditional Chinese Medicine (TCM) and others to pick up the new leadership mantle and carry out needed change for a healthier society.

My appreciation also extends to both my children, Michael and Darren Guarnaccia for their forever understanding, kindness and love for a mother who does not always follow the usual route in life and sometimes breaks the rules.

My final thanks and very deep appreciation is to Sarah for her love and support during the entire book writing process; you know exactly what writing is about.

INTRODUCTION

❧

Teachings come from the women, all the teachings.
All the teachings come from the woman. The devastation of these
governments and all these countries is because they put women
down. Put the women down, your place is not going to work.
When you honor women it's going to work.
~Cecilia Mitchell (a Mohawk elder) from Wisdom Daughters

*W*omen have been doing healing work for thousands of years. Healing is women's innate nature. What I share with you in this book is certainly not new. However, what I offer is a fresh perspective as well as a deeper look into how a very old system of medicine can be given new life. The timing right now is perfect. Women are emerging from silence. My deepest desire is to see woman's way of healing honored. This book is written for my sisters in the healing arts and women who care for others: mothers, grandmothers, aunties, sisters — all of us women!

Woman has been at the forefront of healing since time began, even as she birthed her first child. Her knowledge of healing runs deep. Now, as I step into my fiftieth year of healing work, from my beginnings as a young nurse in New York City, many ideas have revealed themselves to me. These ideas are thoughts and expressions that have come from many years of collected observation. As a nurse that is what I was trained to do — observe the patient, the situation, and the outcome.

Finally, my words reflect what I have witnessed and ruminated on over many years of an exciting and ever changing medical career. As a health care provider, I have observed a dominant western health care system grow stronger. The roles of pharmaceuticals have become a priority in every-day medical decisions, and technological diagnoses and treatment have become increasingly important. Doctors and nurses have forgotten how to touch their patients' bodies, and equally important, how to touch their hearts. Concurrently I have observed the rate of chronic illnesses increase even as the *quality* of life decreases. Is it worth extending life when we fail to take into consideration the quality and richness of that life?

Medicine has an intriguing history, with many twists and turns over the last two millennia. Taking care of the sick was the responsibility of those who had the skills, knowledge, but later this shifted to those with education, and power. Originally, healers were primarily the women of the household, extended family members, or village elders. More importantly, a woman had healing skills without power or education. She gleaned her knowledge from her grandmothers and often practiced unnoticed or unrecognized for her authentic healing ways.

As I began this project of researching and identifying the women who have made contributions, my disappointment rose. I stood in various libraries and found book upon book telling the history of medicine. Very few were about women nor written by women. Even those few books about women were often written by men. The problem with this is simple: it's just not the same story. Women telling the story (herstory) with their feminine voice view any history, including the history of medicine, very differently from men, and understand it differently.

The time has come to recognize this incongruity in healing, name it, and incorporate balance back into all aspects of medicine. In doing this, we will help people find their wellness. The medical team for the chronically ill individual may include physicians, researchers, bio-technicians, nurses, assistants, energy workers, body workers, acupuncturists, aides, social workers, and spiritual ministers. However in general, medicine as a whole is not well connected within its practice of helping people get well and stay healthy. Medical specialties each have their domains of expertise. Often they fail to connect all the healing aspects for the patient who needs it the most.

When we connect, we heal. The machines and technology alone do not heal us. Instead, it is the often overlooked aspect of our interconnection that does. A medical world that operates as separate compartments, independent of one another, is folly. We depend on one another; even in medicine, it "takes a village."

The truth we often hear in women's stories in medicine is that connection heals. Women know how to connect with one another. That is how I believe we will ultimately heal the planet. Continuing and deepening connections to each other by dropping the false sense of separateness can be a pathway to deeper healing.

As time marches on in this new millennia, we are moving into a new awareness. This consciousness is showing up in gatherings among those who know that the direction the collective world is headed is not the answer for planetary survival. These groups include women and men who can see the common thread of healing, close the chasm, and lead the way up and out of rigid thinking and doing things as they have always been done.

I want to explore with you, the reader, how modern medicine has deep roots in military warfare, and how women have tried successfully and unsuccessfully to bring new balance to that paradigm. This book gives a hopeful view on how we can help change the emphasis on war and triumph associated with disease care, and instead embrace connection and intuition to correct the imbalance found in conventional medical healing.

A new power and consciousness is rising; women are feeling more energized by what continues to be rediscovered around feminine energy. Our female wisdom and knowledge is deeply embedded, but women have found it difficult to speak out. I have swallowed my own voice through fear of reprisal, scorn, or ridicule, too often witnessed in my early nursing career. It is my hope that, by writing this book about and for women healers, current and future women in the healing arts will know their full, uncompromised value. There is no second place. Within the realm of wisdom and energy, women have valuable and vital input for the health of this planet. Within deep places like the womb, creation begins; and it can and will continue to flourish with recognition and accolade. As we own this mystery side within and communicate with one another, we can create healing energy, together revealing our true innate nature.

The purpose of this book is to hold a place of honor for woman's contributions. Whether you practice in the healing arts, are a woman raising a family, or are a woman out in the work world, this speaks to you. To find balance within ourselves, in life, and on this planet, it is necessary to hold masculine and feminine healing energies in balance. I explore with the reader the healing arts of western medicine and give my perspective on what is missing in the dominant medical practice. I feel it is important to discuss my experiences as a medical professional, since the current medical model has forgotten to honor the feminine side of medicine. Many wonderful women in the healing arts have contributed tremendously to the healing of humankind. They are relatively unknown, so I want to bring them into the light.

Additionally, I hope to inspire women of all backgrounds to realize their innate energies and power. Our healing powers come from within, not from a medicine bottle or a physician's advice. Every woman who studies and practices any form of medicine needs to know she carries her ancestors' work forward.

Authors David Perlmutter, MD, and Alberto Villoldo, PhD, write about how every cell's mitochondria is carried forward by the female. These authors named it the "feminine life force."[1] We carry the energy of our great grandmothers' cells and pass it on to our future progeny. It is through this idea that I write about a health care system in desperate need of major help.

We need to think of each other as one: one planet, one consciousness, caring more deeply and connecting with each other as one. It is the only thing that makes sense.

I now practice a nurturing holistic form of medicine called naturopathic medicine, after attending a four-year medical school[2] and completing a doctorate in natural medicine in 1990. Learning these natural healing modalities launched me into my second medical career. This work allows me to create a partnership with my clients in their quest for health and wellness.

This quote from Alan Cohen clearly speaks to me: "The power of the heart goes far beyond feeling and emotion; in the heart lies great wisdom and peace."[3]

I am following my heart.

Pamela Sky Jeanne, ND

CHAPTER 1

Caring Through The Ages

~⚬~

Our bodies communicate to us clearly and specifically,
if we are willing to listen.
~Shakti Gawain

Shakti Gawain's quote shows her understanding of what female healers of centuries past have known: health requires intuition and a sense of what heals not just the body but also the mind, heart, and soul. Through stages of development, through the inevitable ebb and flow of life and its circumstances, health is continually changing. The feminine gifts of intuition and connection carry with them the power not only to understand and empathize, but also to revitalize and heal.

This wisdom wasn't granted to women. It wasn't bestowed on females in the 20th century along with the right to vote. It has simply always been. In fact, it was far more highly regarded in ancient times than in our current lifetimes. Certainly there is a growing and resurgent respect for healing wisdom, but to appreciate its scope, we must take a closer look at healing. This book explores women's deep affinity with healing. As I connect the traits women bring to the medical paradigm, you will come to know what I have observed in my last 50 years. My exposure to medicine has been in the proverbial medical "trenches", not in research or academia. In my work I have held many hands and comforted many hearts.

Divine Female Healers of Antiquity

In cultures around the globe, women held positions of reverence and power within their families, tribes, and clans long before recorded history. The term "Mother Earth" isn't just a catch phrase. It is a testament to yin energy, known as the creative, sustaining, healing power of the universal feminine. In fact, the role of feminine energy in healing is so embedded in ancient cultures that it is firmly intertwined with mythology and reality, exactly where it belongs because it honors wholeness.

Archaeological finds have revealed highly developed civilizations among people of Mesopotamia, Egypt, and Greece as far back as the second millennium BC, including evidence that both women and men were respected practitioners of medicine. In the grave of Queen Shubad of Ur (3500 B.C.), researchers have found prescriptions for easing pain, along with surgical instruments of flint and bronze. Several Egyptian queens were renowned for healing, including Queen Mentuhutep (2300 B.C.), whose grave held a large cedar chest containing alabaster jars of ointments, tinctures, measuring spoons, and dried herbs.[4]

The people of Egypt worshipped the goddess Sekhmet, an important icon of power; her name translates to "might and terror." Sekhmet was seen variously as the bringer of diseases, the provider of cures, the avenger of wrongs. She was also called the Scarlet Lady, a reference to blood: she was a special goddess for women, ruling over menstruation. During the Middle Kingdom (2055-1650 BC), she became synonymous with physicians and surgeons. At that time, many members of Sekhmet's priesthood held the same status as physicians.[5]

In Ancient Greece, women were often well known as herbalists and healers. Homer's *The Iliad* and *The Odyssey* substantiates this fact. Agamede cared for the wounded and dying of the Greek and Trojan armies in the Trojan War,[6] and Polydamna, "one who subdues disease," dispensed herbs and understood the medicinal use of plants.[7]

Again in Greek history, Artemisia of Caria, fifth century B.C., a medical student and botanist who gave her name to the Artemisia genus of plants, was credited with knowing every herb used in medicine. Over time, though, a more patriarchal system of government and politics developed in Greece, and women were increasingly sidelined in every aspect of public life, including medicine.

However, Agnodice, an Athenian woman who wanted to become a doctor in the fourth century B.C., was determined to make strides. She was able to receive medical training only by disguising herself as a man. Once established as a physician, but still disguising herself, her feminine, intuitive means of practice earned her a large following. Unfortunately, it also garnered the jealousy of her male colleagues. When other physicians discovered her true female identity, Agnodice faced the death penalty for practicing medicine. What saved her were her female patients who threatened mass suicide if she were not allowed to treat them. The law was changed to allow "gentlewomen" to become doctors as long as they only treated women and children. Ancient Greece set a vital precedent for all female healers who followed Agnodice.[8]

The art and science of gynecology made huge strides with the work of Aspasia, a Greco-Roman woman of the first century A.D. She devised surgical procedures to treat tumors, peritonitis, fibroids, and varicose veins, and wrote a classic text on gynecology that remained the standard for nearly one thousand years. It included specifics for special prenatal diets and exercise, and descriptions of how to prepare herbal tampons for contraception. Although these accounts are of specific women, in general, the fabled village wise woman—sometimes referred to as a witch—held a place of honor among her people. She carried the traditions of her ancestors and passed them onto her daughters and granddaughters. Assisting from birth to death, she was revered for her skill, wisdom, and knowledge.

It is true that throughout history, some women have held positions of power and received educations, particularly if they belonged to the aristocratic class or lived a religious life. However, their numbers were very small. Opportunities for women in the healing practices were more limited in urban than in rural areas, where few physicians practiced.

Peasants and villagers used common remedies, including charms, spells and potions, with great—and recorded—success. Meanwhile, the privileged classes had access to the scientific knowledge and medical practices of their time, which increasingly encroached on traditional healing methods. An interesting paradox of higher learning is that many medical treatments originated from the empirical methods of the peasant population. The rise of scientific medicine began in the 17th and 18th centuries during which time the scientific community had disdain for healers' experimental methods. Yet ironically, modern scientific research relies on trial-and-error experimentation. Early healers learned what did and did not work for their patients, discarded what didn't work, and passed down what did work to succeeding generations. The female healer learned and practiced what worked. Note: during this period of time, the "regular" doctors' remedies such has blood-letting, heavy metals like mercury, and cathartics were harsh and often fatal treatments.[9] Common people were also reluctant to use these medical treatments, preferring the herbal remedies.

Women collected herbs and created recipes for treating diseases. Oftentimes, especially for the sick and poor, the only affordable practitioner was the "old wife" of the community. In this era of oral history, these wise women told stories about the herbal potions they used. Some writings capture these as "old wives' tales."

As these herbs became part of the early medicines and drugs that educated doctors used, eventually a pharmacopoeia emerged describing the uses and actions of herbs. To gain control of this knowledge, medical orthodoxy discredited old wives' tales that dealt with herbal remedies.[10]

Evidence of women healers in history books or current medical texts and education is scant at best; yet there is clear reverence for feminine power in ancient cultures, apparent in essential words and names. The word "hygiene," for example, comes from Hygeia, the Goddess of Good Health, one of the daughters of the Earth mother Rhea. (She comes from the Asclepius family in Greek mythology) We know a panacea as a "cure all," but it was first the name of Rhea's twin sister. The Hippocratic Oath, to which all doctors pledge themselves, uses both of those terms. The Sanskrit word media, meaning feminine wisdom, is the root word of "medicine" as well as the names of goddesses associated with healing such as Medea and Medusa.[11]

The Power to Name

With the rise of the Christian era came the decline of the presence of women in the healing arts. Over several centuries, women's participation in medical practices was held in disregard, if not with downright suspicion. Nearly all formal schooling for women was under the auspices of the Catholic church.[12] Most women learned—as they always had—through empirical methods and traditions passing on orally, largely unwritten, from grandmother to mother to daughter. Women's voices were hushed to whispers, shared in each other's safety and confidence, while men received formal medical training.

Adrienne Rich says, "Where language and naming are power, silence is oppression, is violence."[13]

This is a reference to Adamic Tradition, which holds that (s)he who holds the power to name and delineate holds a more general power. This authority is frequently wielded with disregard, if not downright vengeance, for those with lesser power or those from whom power has been taken. With the increased influence of the Adamic Tradition came the loss of recorded healing traditions, methods, cures, and research. As religious power was taken by the few, so was medical power and thus came the rise of scientific elitism. Healing practices that had once been intuitive, personal, and hands-on evolved into the scientific realm dominated by theory and scientific proof, as the only acceptable means of healing.

This phenomenon occurred over time, of course. But increasingly, physicians used erudite medical terminology while expressing mistrust and disdain for the intuitive and/or empirical methods so long employed by women healers. As science developed, the disdain for empirical methods grew. A woman who did not have the same education as men relied on her working knowledge. During this time men were trained in scientific methodology and disregarded any health related methods not proven by science. Illnesses, maladies—mental, physical, emotional, and spiritual—were categorized and specifically termed. Latin or Greek root derivative prefixes and suffixes were assigned to specific "symptoms"; treatments were assigned to each malady. The word "gastritis", for example, comes from the Greek root word "gastro," meaning stomach, and "itis," meaning inflammation. To the average person—whether in 210 A.D. or 2010 A.D.—medical language is difficult to understand. It kept (and keeps) the doctor in charge by using a language only professionals speak. Medical elitism contributed to the separation of doctor and patient, establishing and maintaining the doctor's control. Slowly but surely, the "power" to heal moved from a joint effort of patient and healer to something controlled by the healer or doctor and delivered to the patient.

When people paid the village wise woman for her medicine, the community doctor's earnings diminished, eventually leading to the continued decline of women in the healer's role. Her practices were seen as unreliable and only scientific medicine was of value. Old wives' tales weren't discarded, however. Instead, male healers added the vital knowledge to their own practices, often assigning scientific names to the remedies and the illnesses they treated. Thus, politics, economics, and class influenced women's status in practicing medicine.

The loss of longstanding traditions of the female healer, which were incorporated by the male counterpart, is not well documented. Mary Chamberlain states, "The old wives' tale should be heard, not only to redress a historical imbalance, but also for the insights it may now throw on modern medical practices."[14]

Cultural practices surrounding childbirth are further examples of the changes that medical elitism imposed on women. According to archaeological records that span cultures around the world, for centuries birth was simply women's sphere. Period. Pregnancy was not considered a medical condition; birthing was not something for which a woman needed "treatment." Women helped women through pregnancy, labor, and delivery. It was a natural occurrence; women knew instinctively how to encourage natural birth using hands-on techniques, herbs, and nutrition. Women knew to employ gravity for assistance during birth, using the traditional squatting position for delivery.

However, childbirth underwent a long-lasting change in the 1600's, when Louis XIV insisted on viewing the birth of his mistress's baby. He instructed the attending physician to have the woman lie down, while the king hid behind a curtain to watch the process. You need only stroll through a labor and delivery ward at most western medical centers to see that this one incident changed the birth process for millions of women. The supine position became standard practice because the king's physician was able to view his patient's body in a new way. Subsequently he taught this technique to his medical colleagues.

There is no scientific proof that supine birthing is superior to squat birthing, but for almost 350 years, babies under the care of the medical establishment have been birthed in this manner. This unnatural birth process often resulted in the need for medical intervention, leading to a higher infant and maternal mortality rate. One example is the ever-increasing rate of cesarean sections. Statistics bear out that babies born in non-medical settings require fewer medical intervention.[15]

When men became medically involved with pregnancy and childbirth, they claimed that because they were formally educated, male midwives knew more about birthing processes than women practitioners: studying the human body gave trained physicians greater knowledge to assure a *good* birth. Doctors assured mothers that earlier intervention could save infant lives. However, current statistics show the US has higher maternal and infant mortality rates than several other countries in the world, 6.14/1000 births. This is higher than Italy, Hungary, Greece, or Cuba![16] Interventions in the birth process based solely on scientific methods create an imbalance or sometimes poorer birth outcomes. In the cases of birth, infant health, and rate of autism, the US, seen as a leader in scientific advances, is failing to achieve the health of its people.

The Standouts

With the predominance of men in obstetrics, some female practitioners either remained below the radar of the powers-that-be or just downright resisted them. Given the energy necessary to keep the feminine flame alive and well in the healing arts, even in the twenty-first century, one has to marvel at the focus, determination, and chutzpah it took for the two thousand years before a woman was ever called a suffragette. Thankfully, there were women with that degree of perseverance and confidence in their skills and knowledge.

Trotula of Salerno is a fine example of such a woman. Although her male counterparts discredited her, she contributed great scholarly works on women's anatomy and physiology. She trained at the University of Salerno, one of the few places women could study in the eleventh century A.D. Details of her life are scarce; however, she authored several medical books, and it is claimed she was a department chair at the University. While medical authorities were critical of her prolific writings, three texts survive and are credited to her: *Diseases of Women*, *Treatments for Women*, and *Women's Cosmetics*. The writings of this trailblazing woman were collected and edited over the next few centuries as they passed through the hands of many subsequent "authors" who claimed credit for her work. *The Trotula*, as the three combined texts became known, is divided into twenty-seven sections and focuses on problems with menstruation and childbirth. It is still well recognized as one of Europe's most important medical texts on women's health.[17]

Hildegard of Bingen was a twelfth century nun, a respected Christian mystic, another prolific writer, and a powerful woman ahead of her time. She wrote music and books on herbal medicine and, most importantly, on the physiology of the human body. As a Benedictine nun, she was cloistered for the first half of her life. In the next 35 years she became a visionary prophet and wrote volumes of books on many subjects.[18] Her texts on the care of the human body revealed herbal remedies and nutritional advice still practiced today as "Hildegard's Medicine."[19] She is still revered for her holistic and natural view of healing.

Women were the keepers of cultural traditions in some Native American cultures, as well. The Iroquois, for example, were historically matriarchal. Women were responsible for defining the political, social, spiritual, economic, and health norms of the tribe. While tribal leaders were men, it was the Clan Mothers who nominated and elected them and retained the power to remove them from their positions. Women ensured males fulfilled their leadership responsibilities. Iroquois women enjoyed social equality and respect, and were credited with the intuitive, healing knowledge that kept clans cohesive and thriving.

The Vanished, the Forgotten, and the Disappeared

To do full justice to all of history's remarkable women healers would take volumes of books, not just a small section in a single chapter. For a myriad of reasons, male practitioners have taken extreme measures to discredit, disable, and disguise woman's work, her practice of healing and her power of connection.

The years from 1300 to 1700 saw staggering numbers of women and their healing practices annihilated. An inquisition spanning those four hundred years focused on both women and men accused of heresy, opposing the prevailing church teachings. In small villages, often women were the only practitioners treating the physically and mentally ill with herbs, spells, and incantations. The purge of these women and their "suspicious" practices saw an estimated over 100,000 up to nine million (figures vary from different sources) people, mostly women (80%), executed for practicing their "craft" which was outside the Christian church's teachings and beliefs.[20] We will never know the exact number, but the effect was indelible. This four-century siege delivered a clear message. Women became powerless and came to accept the second-place status to which they were relegated. In fear for their lives, female healers and those that relied on them remained "underground." Speaking out and becoming educated remained available only for privileged women of the aristocratic ranks.

Not all women healers of note met such drastic fates. For most, the violence they experienced was more emotional and psychological than physical. It was subtler and, some would argue, even more insidious. A slap across the face leaves a red mark, a sign of violation. An assault to the soul or the psyche, however, can leave a trail of doubt and fear that still has an effect on women today.

Blazing a Trail

The collective voice of women healers speaks to us of health and healing for people of all genders, sexualities, classes, and races. Its familiar tone and language graces our ears more clearly with each accomplishment reached, moving women healers closer to a position of well-deserved honor.

To fully appreciate and embrace the promise of balanced healthcare, it is crucial to understand the rise and fall of women's value in every aspect. As members of families, villages, tribes, and clans, women's roles—and lack thereof—have a deep and reverberating impact on the world. The eroding of the feminine position has affected all of humankind and the evolution of healthcare. Feminine contributions and influences on shaping medical practice are poorly understood, as is the lingering contemporary imbalance of "power."

In *Women Healers*, Elisabeth Brooke writes that women have been doctors and were considered natural healers. We remember women who prevailed under the thumb of their class, like Florence Nightingale. Women who were controversial, though, are barely mentioned in history books. It is time to fully celebrate and embrace the feminine side of healing once again.

21ˢᵗ Century Tale

Pamela

"What about all the women?" I asked the professor from my seat in the lecture hall. I felt the eyes of my fellow students turn to me. The room fell silent for an uncomfortably long time until Professor Collins finally responded. "I have no explanation for it, Pamela."

It was the middle of my first year of medical school and I had heard ten weeks of historical lectures on medicine, keeping the faith that some glorious mention of at least one influential woman was just around the corner. In fact, as each week went by, I reassured myself that Professor Collins was saving up all the information on women and planning to devote one entire lecture to it. Suddenly, though, there I was at the close of the final lecture with copious notes on the history of male contributions to medicine. I, along with my classmates, had only half of the story. I was stunned that women's contributions were unacknowledged. If the history of women was not taught at this progressive natural medical college, I knew it was surely not included in mainstream medical education for physicians.

"There have been many female contributors to medicine," I said to Professor Collins, "but there was no mention of any female physicians, scientists, or lay healers in this course." Collins looked at me quizzically for a moment. I knew I had his attention. He subsequently invited me to join him the following years as a guest lecturer to present insights into woman's contributions to the evolution of medicine. I was thrilled to give these guest lectures and continued to do so for four years. Still, as I moved into my career, I saw on a daily basis how far we had to go for women's participation in healing to be acknowledged, respected, and honored.

❧

CHAPTER 2

Balance in Medicine

~ⓖ~

*"The principle of yin and yang is the foundation
of the entire universe."*
~Yellow Emperor Huang Di

"Information is NOT knowledge."
~ Albert Einstein

The concept of yin and yang balance is not common
in western medical thought. It is part of Chinese culture, the
cornerstone of science, philosophy, and medicine since
before the Christian era.[21] Simply put, yin and yang is a way
of describing the flow of life, energy, and, ultimately, balance.

The key here is balance. In Chinese society understanding yin and yang is the basis for understanding life, from
birth to death, and for defining states of health and disease.
Along life's journey, yin and yang energies ebb and flow in a
constant quest for balance. The basis of the 5000-year-old
principle is that everything and everyone—whether a physical
being, an emotional relationship, or an inanimate corporation—is comprised both of yin (or feminine) and yang (or
masculine) qualities. Yin qualities are slow, soft, yielding,

diffuse, cold, wet, or tranquil. It is associated with water, earth, the moon, femininity, and nighttime. Yang qualities, on the other hand, are fast, hard, solid, focused, hot, dry, or aggressive. It is associated with fire, sky, the sun, masculinity, and daytime. Everyone and everything we know operates *optimally* only when both sides are in balance.

Yin and yang qualities are not static. A balance scale can be a metaphor for one's physical, mental, and emotional self, with yin on one side and yang on the other; but realize that the scale is one integral whole, constantly moving within one being. The balance between the two forces changes constantly depending on a great number of factors: nutrition, stress, joy, grief, harmony...the list goes on. Consciously or subconsciously, we call on our own unique yin/yang in an effort to create balance in our physical beings, our environments, and our lives.

A woman is not 100% yielding and passive in every circumstance at all times. Similarly, no man is 100% aggressive and authoritarian. If either of these traits is excessively dominant in a person for any length of time, it indicates an imbalance of some sort, be it at work, in relationships, or in one's health. Lack of balance causes disharmony and disease. We all know of people whose health has suffered—even to the point of death—after prolonged periods of stress. When and how did these people become out of balance? And, more importantly, how have they brought themselves back into balance?

American writer and author Frank Herbert once said, "There's no secret to balance. You just have to feel the waves." States of imbalance cause reactions, a push and pull, a give and take, in a person or a thing. Disharmony and imbalance of our energies cause disease, by being dominated by one wave instead of a balance of both—like the tide moving in and then moving out. In the third century B.C.E., the Yellow Emperor Huang Di said it well, and we are finally starting to listen. He said, "The principle of yin and yang is the foundation of the entire universe. It underlies everything in creation. It brings about the development of parenthood; it is the root and source of life and death. It is found with the temples of the gods."[22]

We must access both our masculine and feminine sides. And we must embrace both of them to affect our own healing. Harmony and balance wait for us to claim them. And when we heal ourselves, we contribute toward healing the world around us.

A Harmonious Blend

To understand the journey from sickness to health, consider yin and yang as harmonious opposites. From this perspective, the body is yin and yang at the same time. Illnesses occur if there is too much or too little of either yin or yang. Nothing is purely yin or purely yang. For example, something can be primarily yin, but also have yang qualities. Consider water temperature. Water can be neutral ("room temperature"), a little warm, a little cool, or extremely hot or cold. Thinking of yin as cool and yang as warm, the parallels are striking. Very hot or very cold water can be detrimental, while a neutral temperature can be soothing and calming. The balanced combination of hot and cold—a blending of opposites—is ideal.

On t-shirts, brochures, billboards, and menus, this symbol, the Taijitu, is the depiction of yin and yang. Taijitu literally translates to "diagram of the supreme ultimate." For health and healthcare, it is the perfect visual symbol for homeostasis, or the tendency for established systems to maintain stability. The most significant thing about the Taijitu

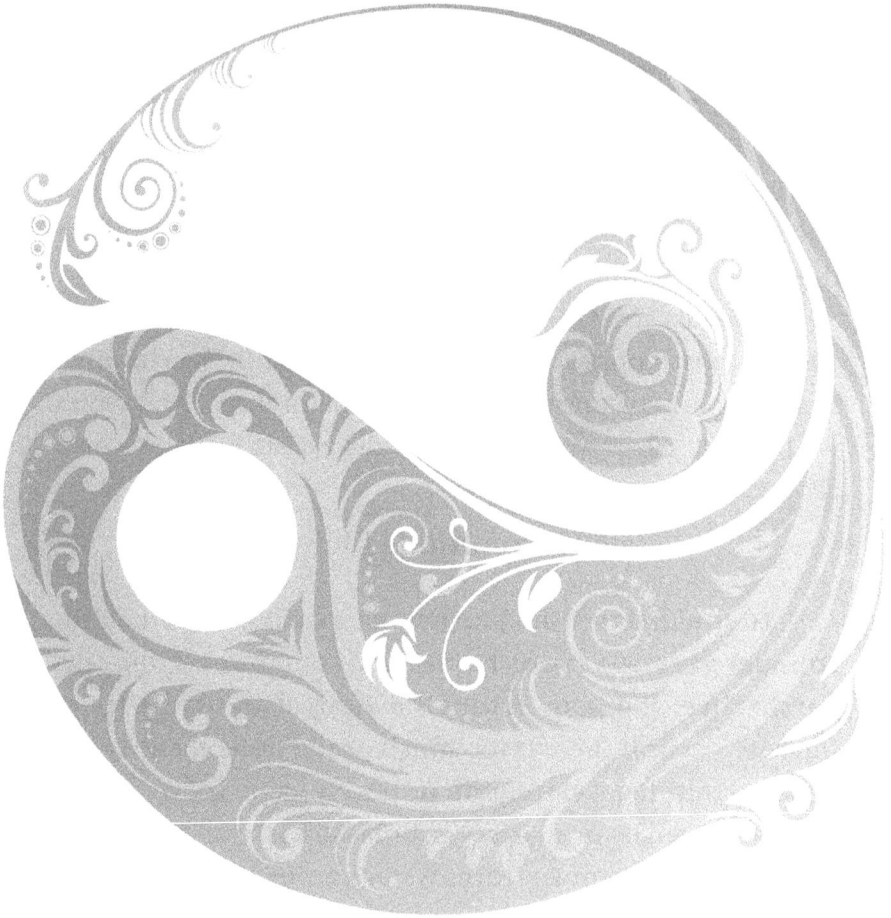

symbol is that the two components do not simply stand next to one another, divided by a straight line. They blend into one another, forming a perfect, never-ending circle, one half intrinsically part of the other. Yin and yang are opposites, that is true, but each is also one-part of a whole. Fully dependent, they need each other to be complete. This concept is basic to understanding balance and harmony. An excess or lack of one or the other will eventually, inevitably, lead to illness of the mind, body, or both. That certain groups of people currently experience increasing rates of illness and earlier morbidity (disease) speaks to the dominance of yang in our western culture. Current yang style medicine practices can stop disease symptoms very well but more people are living longer with chronic degenerative, debilitating diseases. Without the balance of yin qualities in medical practice we do not witness people recovering from illnesses, but rather the illness is merely managed.

Beyond the Battle Between Good and Evil

Western language is inept at explaining such ethereal aspects of life as yin and yang balance. It is easy to see that these relationships are ignored in the hands of western medicine providers. What is missing is a deeper understanding of how complementary medical therapies can bring balance medical care. Current medical knowledge is research-based. A hypothesis must be proven without a shadow of doubt; experiments must prove the reliability of a scientific theory before it can be accepted. The same treatment must result in a repeatable, exacting, predictable outcome. Using only scientific knowledge to treat a body's imbalance may ignore critical elements of the whole system (body, mind and spirit).

In western healthcare, where descriptions of health actually use the term homeostasis to denote balance, we tend to see and hear discussions of the imbalance itself, but there is little attention paid to what leads to the loss of balance in the first place. The problem is that western science poorly defines balance in reference to health. One of the ways a clinician can assess body balance is to ask how well a patient is sleeping and what kind of daytime energy the patient experiences. Sleep and energy are indicators of a body in balance. Conventional practitioners often miss asking these questions. Young children who are eating and sleeping well have boundless energy. Our adult bodies are designed to produce enough energy for exercising, thinking, working and having fun. This is an example of optimal balance.

For many clinicians, dualities are often seen as mutually exclusive rather than as complementary, as in the earlier example of hot and cold water. Quite different from the eastern perspective, we learn in western culture that right is the opposite of wrong. We emphasize black or white, good or bad, up or down. The operative word here is "or." We are taught that if one aspect is correct, then the opposite aspect must be incorrect. There are many, many more examples of this polarizing belief. As represented in the Taijitu symbol, so called-dualities can actually complement one another, benefiting and balancing the entity as a whole. There is no "or." There is only "and."

This battle of good versus evil appears in stories, movies, and songs throughout western culture. Whether we realize it or not, it is the prevailing Christian-Judeo philosophy; the fixed, finite Ten Commandments infuse and heavily influence our western concept of right and wrong, black and white, cause and effect so replete in our medical system. It has shaped the majority of western civilization's idea of dualism as the existence of two separate things or ideas, not the blending of them.

Precision and narrow parameters certainly have a place in our world. In their absence, a space shuttle launch would be, and has been, disastrous. A military maneuver without tactical exactness is harrowing. In surgery, medical diagnostic procedures, and pharmaceutical dosing, precision is essential to safeguard the patient. When this precision is the main operative in all human healing, though, it has limited usefulness. Preventable disaster occurs when the human is forgotten in favor of the illness and when a patient's emotional, spiritual, and psychic needs are minimized or overlooked altogether. Unlike a jet or a space shuttle, a human is not a piece of machinery on a precisely charted yang-style course.

An Integrated Dance

The feminine, or yin, qualities of medicine are important in the treatment of the ill. These qualities include nurturing. The yin side is not *the* most important element, but without it, a huge void is left in moving toward wellness. True healing and recovery require balance; some equate this as mind-body-spirit wholeness. And in the imbalance within the male-dominated profession, the feminine voice and ideas have been lost. *Her* value and *her* ideas have gone unrecognized and forgotten.

The ideal of balance is not just a matter of "hot and cold makes warm", but a complex interplay of each cell's physical activity. When illness sets in, all the factors involved with getting well add to the mix. These factors may include the ill person's concerns about being taken care of (or not wanting to be), pain (control of and relief from), fatigue, memory loss, clarity of mind, anxiousness of being a burden, and feeling hopeless of ever being well. Positive emotions can help in the healing process; negative emotions can hinder the return to a state of balanced health.

The yin and yang charts below show how each opposite human quality can operate alone or as part of the other. We actually do operate on both sides of the spectrum in a complex and beautiful dance, as first one side leads and then the other, at different times in our lives. A dance occurs when they alternate between leading and following.

QUALITIES OF THE MIND	
YANG	**YIN**
Rational	Irrational
Form	Process
Intellect	Intuition
Knowledge	Wisdom
Decisive	Flexible
Analysis	Synthesis
Linear	Circular
Mastery	Mystery
Proactive	Reactive
Extroverted	Introverted

QUALITIES OF THE HEART	
YANG	**YIN**
Curing	Caring
Light	Dark
Sun	Moon
Giving	Receiving
Unique	Unity
Competition	Collaboration
How	Why
Focus	Perspective
Open	Closed

QUALITIES OF THE SPIRIT	
YANG	**YIN**
Physical world	Invisible realm
Sky	Earth
Power	Compassion
Outside	Inside
Demanding	Yielding
All-knowing	Reflective
External/Public	Internal/Private
Religion	Spirit

Yin and Yang in the Body

Traditional Chinese Medicine, and specifically acupuncture, works to restore a healthy yin and yang balance. A clinical example of a liver imbalance is a person who has headaches, a flushed face, and feelings of anger. The yin and yang relationship may be 70% yang and 30% yin, leading to excessive yang symptoms.

Needle acupuncture has been successful for 2,000 years.[23] Yet, before 1972, the western medical perspective said this form of diagnosis and treatment was unscientific and bordered on voodoo medicine. Eventually, Chinese doctors were able to show western doctors the power of acupuncture by performing surgical procedures using acupuncture needles in place of western anesthetics. Studies began to appear everywhere on the role of endorphins and enkephalins, (tiny prostaglandins produced within the body), substances that are associated with pain relief. Once there was a "scientific" explanation of pain relief via the prostaglandin system, the door opened wide to Chinese therapy: pain relief resulted from stimulation with acupuncture needles of the body's meridians. A great weakness of western science is the tendency to reject what is unseen, and that tendency, entrenched in our medical world, can sometimes work against itself. As the above chart illustrates, dark and light qualities are of equal value, just as are night and day, and power and compassion. The body as a whole does not and cannot function separately in the emotional and physiologic spheres.

Much of western medicine follows an allopathic[24] philosophy based on an idea of mutually exclusive dualities: the physical and the non-physical. Compartmentalized medical practices or subspecialties make this fact quite obvious. Physicians often view and treat a person with a physical disease without considering their emotions and/or spirituality. Physicians may become so specialized in their fields of medicine that they are reluctant to treat another part of the body.

In Chinese medical practices, history indicates a respect for yin. Although most women in early Chinese culture were subjugated to male power, Charlotte Furth writes in *A Flourishing Yin* that women held status in the obstetric realm. Children owed respect to the woman who gave them life and care in their young years; therefore, obstetrics was a natural path for a woman interested in medicine. Language offers another significant perceptual difference in the two cultures. The definition of our English word "body" is sorely limited. When we hear the word, we tend to think of the physical form. In comparison, the Chinese word "shen" means "body/person" and takes into account the entire being including its spirit. In ancient Chinese medical writings, shen encompassed the psyche, the emotions, and the physical form, treating body-mind as one entity.[25] It seems the west has much to learn, and much more to embrace, about the entirety of ourselves as human beings.

Contemporary Women Balancing Yin and Yang

Many women, through either desire or necessity, take the healthcare of loved ones into their own hands. Among the Saraguro Indians in the southern highland of Ecuador, for instance, women who are mothers and heads of households provide extraordinary home health care, despite the availability of modern medicine in urban centers. These women balance the available yang in the medical facilities with their yin practice of in-home health care. Inspired by that example, Professor Ruthbeth Finerman, a noted medical anthropologist, conducted a twelve-month survey that revealed that 86% of family illness was treated by women's home remedies. "Cross cultural studies show that women and in particular female heads of household represent a major source of therapeutic assistance in many societies," says Finerman.[26] We see this truth everywhere from remote villages to suburban naturopathic clinics to the aisles of home remedies in urban natural food markets.

Carol Shepherd Mc Clain, PhD, has also done extensive research in medical anthropology. She weighs the controversy of whether home remedies are too simplistic in her book, *Women as Healers*, where she cites numerous indigenous cultures using combination therapies with considerable efficacy; these include laying on of hands, herbal remedies, poultices, and juices. While the mysterious effectiveness of many of these remedies defies scientific explanation, the fact remains that such alternative therapies work or they wouldn't have crossed over cultural boundaries and survived extensive timelines. Women know it, and use them to heal their families.

Another group of healers is the curanderas. These women retain and use healing techniques passed down from the Mayans and Incas. With a focus on spiritual techniques and channeling the energies of their patients, as well as God, angels, and beings of light, these women bring physical, mental, and emotional healing to their patients. There are three types of curanderas: sobaderosas or bone and muscle therapists; parteras or midwives and herbalists.[27] Dr. Clarissa Pinkola Estes, author of the bestseller *Women Who Run With the Wolves*, is among the many who applaud the work of the curanderas.

Midwives, doulas, and lactation educators are shining

examples of the blending of yin and yang. Midwives provide alternatives to the traditional obstetrician-assisted pregnancy and birth. Doulas, from an ancient Greek word that literally means "mother's slave," are professionally trained and certified pregnancy and childbirth assistants. DONA (Doulas of North America) describes a doula as one who "provides continuous physical, emotional and informational support to the mother before, during and just after birth; or who provides emotional and practical support during the postpartum period." Studies show that when doulas assist in birth, labors are shorter with fewer complications and babies are healthier and breastfeed more easily than conventional hospital births.[28]

Women in these professions, and the women and men who pay for their services, represent the harmonious blend of yin and yang. They are found everywhere from private homes to birthing centers to hospitals, alongside western medicine that is available if and when necessary.

Marie is a long-time doula who has helped hundreds of women to achieve the childbirth experiences they desired in hospitals. In her experience, "Being in a traditional setting and having both an obstetrician and a doula is the best of both worlds for a lot of women." This complementary duality is yin balancing yang.

Like the "old wives", healers in smaller regions or urban apartment blocks or suburban cul-de-sacs use spiritual as well as physical remedies, and that includes good old TLC. Dr. McClain gives a good example in what she calls the "local-level healer." "These healers translate, mediate, and perpetuate traditional medical knowledge, linking it with respected social traditions in interaction with patients and patients' families. They conceptualize allopathic, Ayurvedic,

Buddhism, and exorcism in a single framework that also includes daily prescriptions of cleanliness, good nutrition, proper social relations, environmental sanitation and the like, all viewed as crucial to the maintenance of health."[29] While Dr. McClain was discussing a particular study, we could expand the terms she uses, to see that she is talking about mothers, acupuncturists, school nurses, cranio-sacral healers, enlightened MDs, and others who focus on the whole person.

Flowing into Balance

The current western medical system is an example of yin and yang imbalance that needs to be set right. Many people report dissatisfaction with the care they receive in the current model. Five- to seven-minute visits with a medical provider, very short hospitalizations for complex procedures, same-day surgeries, and overmedicating with pharmaceutical drugs are but a few of the common complaints that practitioners in alternative fields hear.

Some critics call our "health care" system a disease care system. Its focus is to manage diseases caused by the loss of health balance. Many people, myself included, believe that conventional medicine has lost sight of what health looks like. Too many of its practitioners are unaware of, and do not lead, a truly healthful lifestyle. How can so-called health care providers help patients live healthfully if they themselves cannot? Conventional medical, osteopathic, and nursing programs primarily teach pathology and disease recognition (diagnosis). This method is helpful for those individuals who have lost their health balance. At this point it is critical to "fix" the problem so further body damage is avoided. But that's only half of the equation; here is where balance is essential. If the practitioner and the patient don't seek that balance point, homeostasis in many cases may be restored only by radical treatments such as pharmaceutical drugs, chemotherapy, radiation, and/or surgery. These treatments are yang-based—fast, physical, active, aggressive, and powerful.

In these situations, the yang approach addresses the immediate need, but the body can't be restored to full, optimum health without attending the yin side. The yin brings caring, receiving, absorbing, and accepting: the quiet side of healing. In this palette of healing components, nutrition is essential. For example, proper nutrition and high-quality, precisely prescribed nutritional supplements can not only halt a pre-diabetic state, but can actually reverse it. Conventional practitioners, however, mainly help people control and manage their disease, but doing so is not curative. Disease management is palliative (meaning eased or lessened without curing), not healing. A hospital may be an appropriate place for a good deal of disease care, but when are people, not merely patients, given the tools, support, and time to heal truly and completely?

21st Century Tale

Vaughn

Vaughn retired from his fast-paced urban life to the quiet of northern Idaho. He expected to ease into tranquility. Much to his dismay, his days became filled with anxiety and mounting health issues. When he finally visited an MD in the nearest town, he was pleasantly surprised. Vaughn said he nearly fell off of the exam table when the young doctor, in his mid-30's, set down his clipboard and pen, leaned on the table, and inquired about his patient's stress-level and nutrition. He also asked if Vaughn had any family in the area with whom he spent quality time. The doctor ordered a full-spectrum of blood tests and subsequently referred his patient to a trusted chiropractor/naturopath who could help turn around the early signs of pre-diabetes and pancreatitis with nutritional supplements and dietary changes. Six months later, Vaughn's objective health issues had resolved and he had alleviated some stress by taking a volunteer position at the local farmer's market, thanks to the doctor's connection there. Now, this is an example of yin and yang balance. Despite the grave imbalance in our healthcare system, there are still many opportunities to witness positive changes happening all around.

❧

A Voice in the Dark

Alice Hamilton MD (1868-1970) was a standout of her era. As a woman in the emerging field of medicine, she pioneered changes for the poor unskilled worker. The industrial revolution was in full swing in the late nineteenth and early twentieth century when this young MD began practicing. She found there were masses of workers incapacitated by the dangerous chemicals they worked with, chemicals that caused chronic illness and death. These workers included miners, steel and metal workers, and those exposed to carbon monoxide fumes and other inhalants. The work of Dr. Hamilton started a new revolution, a movement to protect the industrial worker from the toxicity of his work environment. It was through her diligent observation, treatment, recording and reporting of these dangers faced by the common worker that she helped create safer working conditions and was responsible for the birth of a worker's compensation movement in Illinois, the first in the country. Her findings were so scientifically persuasive that they led to sweeping reforms improving the health of workers. Because she also studied abroad she learned that the US was not paying attention to the health of its industrial workers. Studying the emerging laboratory science of toxicology, she pioneered occupational epidemiology and industrial hygiene in the United States. Literally she helped save thousands of lives. I credit this to her yin sensibilities toward the plight of the poor, voiceless worker.[30]

Awareness from Within

As members of the human race and of any culture, we are easily drawn into the consciousness of the time and place in which we reside. As we live, learn, and interact with family, coworkers, and friends, we take in tremendous amounts of information. What we do with this information can have a direct influence on the balance of our health. We all experience waxing and waning states of health. Through time, we learn what works for us. We learn that coming into balance includes letting go of struggles, resistance, emotional pain, and unkindness that don't serve us well. We innately want balance; we want to feel well, enjoy good energy, and have an inner sense of peace. We want to be happy. Some days we are calm, content, and settled; some days we are frantic, excited, adventuresome, overworked. Here is the fundamental question: can there be balance? At the end of each day we must rest and sleep deeply, but how often does that happen? In western culture, the work ethic often numbs our senses and instincts. How many of our days are spent in happy hours of laughter, rest, and relaxation? In this country and in this century, the common pattern is to do more and more, and have less and less time to dedicate to our families, our friends, our communities, and ourselves. Because awareness is a starting point for any change, we must ask questions. What we internalize will be externalized. Thus balance must first come from within.

Extending this logic to the macrocosm, the world is in a constant state of imbalance. Conflict and unrest between groups of people, countries pitted against one another in a climb for power and control, are indications of an overall yang energy that has led us away from true balance.

21st Century Tale

Pamela

When did I decide to become a nurse? My father decided it for me when I was very young. Programmed to believe that being in service to others was good for me, and because I was told, "You'll always have a job in case something happens to your husband," I dutifully followed the career path designated for me. I applied to and graduated from a nurses training program at Bellevue Hospital Center in NYC. Upon graduation I immediately gravitated to critical care nursing. Staying in this field of work for most of my career as an ICU nurse, I was blindly driven toward becoming a critical care post-operative specialist, an emergency room RN, and eventually a head nurse.

Why did I continue in this over-stimulating, stressful work environment? The work was exhausting and exhilarating at the same time;

I seemed to thrive in it. The stimulus of urgency and rescue was seemingly in my blood. Or was it?

Then one day I awakened! The enlightenment came easily 25 years later during a self-reflective time, as I reviewed my life path. In my quiet introspective session, my mind opened and things got instantly clear. My mother had died unexpectedly by her own hand – suicide. At that time, I was a 5-month-old infant sleeping in the next room. Somewhere, somehow in my subconscious mind it became incomprehensible to me that I was unable to save her. My infant/child mind was frozen with this idea; unconsciously, I was still trying to save my dear mother...and anyone else I possibly could. In every ER trauma/drama I was working through losing a mother who could not be saved.

When this realization came to me, I was done–done working in any urgent or critical medical care, that is. I moved from the yang of my life to the yin, using quiet reflection and an open heart.

I was able to leave a career I had felt compelled to excel in and I have never regretted the decision. I no longer needed this part of me. I now could align my own desires with my truest self and not follow a societal expectation or, worse yet, a less understood and unconscious drive.

Had I continued in that environment, my mental, emotional, and physical health would have been affected. I took further steps in my quest for balance when I decided to return to medical school, eventually graduating from a naturopathic school of medicine. Subsequently I went on to practice the true art of healing.

Countless people have confided in me as a physician how unhappy they are in their marriage, work life, or social life. This aspect of medicine, the yin side, is often minimized or ignored. When a patient suffers from repetitive headaches, a drug or even an herb will relieve the pain in the short term, but will not eliminate the headaches until their cause is addressed. Balance must be restored to the psyche to allow the headaches to abate completely. Many people have sought my help to improve their state of wellness, and the best successes come when underlying causes were acknowledged and treated using counseling, homeopathy, and/or lifestyle and nutritional changes. My life became healthy and whole. Peace and calm became my friends, and I spend my days helping others to achieve similar states in their own lives.

CHAPTER 3

The Womb of Western Medicine

❧

"War is a poor chisel to carve out tomorrow."
~ *Dr. Martin Luther King*

"There are a number of ways to improve progress without resorting to weapons of war."
~ *Cynthia Darlington – Author in* The Female Brain

*M*any of us think of conventional medicine as our safety net. We carry health insurance cards, choose from a list of "preferred providers," have "primary care" physicians, and know that, in the event of illness or accident, a platform of protocols and accepted procedures stands firmly in place. How many times do we hear or say, "You're the doctor," acquiescing to the superior knowledge of the "expert"? We do it because we want resolution of an issue for instance and chronic recurrent problem or a new pain or disability; we place our trust in someone with credentials, hoping they can fix the problem resolving the issue quickly.

We have done the same in times of social upheaval, trusting our leaders to guide us back to safety. In times of war, we hear terms like conquer, fight, win, bravery, invade, orders, ranks, weapons, and overrun to breed courage and hope in our allies and to strike terror in the enemy.

War and Medicine

Where else are these terms part and parcel of everyday language and terminology? How about the "fight" against illness? We "fight cancer," handle the situation "with bravery," follow "doctor's orders" and believe that "with the right weapons, we can beat the illness."

There is good reason that such language appears in a setting so apparently removed from the military. Not long ago, the most intense and widespread medical training occurred not in classrooms, but on battlefields.

Two centuries of American history were dominated by major wars, both on our soil and across the world. The battlefield thus became the classroom for medical practice. The organized structure of the military strongly influenced blood-soaked western medicine.

Thankfully, two events improved conditions for treatment and chances for survival of the wounded: Pasteur's discovery of bacteria and nurses' use of hygienic principles. Prior to the Crimean War, the chief cause of death was infectious diseases that flourished in the unsanitary conditions of the battlefield and poorly constructed medical barracks. In fact, four times more soldiers died from typhus, typhoid fever, cholera, and dysentery than from battle wounds.[31] Diseases that were fatal to injured soldiers spread rapidly at the makeshift hospitals because of overcrowding, defective sewers, and lack of ventilation and running water.

Western medicine made huge strides in technology and scientific knowledge by treating battlefield casualties. Faced with acute traumatic injuries, physicians increased their expertise and honed their surgical skills. War zones provided critical on-the-job training. Medical conditions and, of course, training and preparedness, have improved exponentially since; sadly, in the 21st century we too often treat an ill population like wounded soldiers.

Nursing is considered a noble profession today. Its origin, though, might surprise you. Because the first nurses received little formal training and very low pay, nursing attracted women of the lower socioeconomic classes desiring to help others. Many of the first "nurses" were actually prostitutes that male physicians convinced to help the cause, most notably during the Crimean War in the 19th century. Needless to say, the nursing profession was low on the social hierarchy, a fact emphasized by the doctors of the era.

It wasn't until Florence Nightingale (1820-1910) joined the ranks that the nursing profession, and opinions about it, began to change. Following her groundbreaking and tireless work during the Crimean War, she established her nursing school at St Thomas' Hospital in London in 1860. It was the first secular nursing school in the world. Nurses still take the Nightingale Pledge and the annual International Nurses Day is celebrated worldwide on her birthday. She was called "The Lady With the Lamp" after a newspaper story in *The New York Times* in 1910 recounted her accomplishments.

"The Queen of Nurses" and "The Soldier's Friend" are titles which have stuck to Florence Nightingale since her memorable service in behalf of the wounded and dying in the Crimean war... It was not only in the details of nursing, but in the gentle and watchful care for his comfort that Miss

Nightingale made herself a beautiful memory to the soldier. She lent her aid to the surgeons when strong men turned away in horror, and sustained the courage of the wounded by her appeals to the ties which bound them to home."[32]

Nightingale did more to improve hospital conditions than any other person in history. Her methods were simple: hygiene, sanitation, and clean air. She orchestrated the cleanup of the unkempt, filthy surroundings that housed the fallen soldiers by organizing and educating those who cared for them. She insisted that the hospitals needed clean water and working sewage disposal. In March 1855, six months after Florence Nightingale's arrival, the British government sent out a Sanitary Commission to Scutari to flush sewers, improve ventilation — and save lives.[33]

Nightingale is remembered not only for such achievements, but also for elevating the status of the nursing profession. She contributed much more to the improvement of medicine than is widely recognized. Not only was she a skilled nurse, but she was also a brilliant statistician. This enabled her to monitor the death and recovery rates of the wounded under her care, and to show the impact of the improvements made in the wretched buildings that housed the injured and dying soldiers.[34]

Her statistics showed a decline in the soldiers' death rate from over 40% to less than 5%. Ironically, because she was a woman, she could not sit on the commissions held by the Army to report on her years of findings! However, her work was well known by her allies, and it had a profound effect on the improvement of sanitary conditions in patient care. This ultimately helped to reform the military's care of the wounded. Nightingale's story is a true example of yin medicine.

Female Misalignment

Nightingale died peacefully in her sleep at the ripe old age of 90. Still, somehow, a rumor managed to circulate that she died of syphilis and that she was driven to her work to cover up a covert sexual life style. It is highly unlikely that the vital, hardworking, 90-year-old Nightingale died of debilitating syphilis. The reference to her sexuality may be designed to distract from her life's work, to discredit a great female healer. Time and again this phenomenon has occurred. Women who have made significant contributions to medicine and whose accomplishments have shaped the "early face" of medicine consistently experienced scrutiny and attack.

The pioneering women in medicine persevered with their work, although slandering their professional achievements and publicly questioning their mental and social behavior were effective forms of oppression.

Margaret Sanger's life offers another example of this oppression. Early in the 20th century, she coined the term "birth control", saying that a woman should be "the absolute mistress of her own body." She launched *The Woman Rebel*, an eight-page monthly newsletter promoting contraception. In August 1914, she was indicted for violating US postal obscenity laws, but jumped bail and fled to England under an alias. After she returned, she founded the American Birth Control League in 1921, followed by the first legal birth control clinic staffed entirely by female doctors and social workers in the U.S. In 1923 she formed the National Committee on Federal Legislation for Birth Control, serving as its president until1937, by which time birth control was legal in many states. In 1927, she helped organize the first World Population Conference in Geneva — quite a fitting achievement for a Catholic girl who saw her mother endure 18 pregnancies with no other option.[35]

Sanger was slandered for being married more than once. She was jailed several times, harangued and harassed as a heretic for giving women the rights and means to plan the number of pregnancies their bodies would experience. Opponents described her work as advocating not just birth control, but also women's unwarranted sexual freedom. Like Mary Magdalene (biblically known as a prostitute), a patron of women's spirituality, Margaret Sanger became a victim of the oppressive strategies designed to silence or degrade women.

As we become more knowledgeable of women's great works in medicine, the misjudgments and mistruths about them are hard to ignore. It is my desire to reaffirm the greatness of such women and remember them in the positive frame they so deserve.

Wearing the Chains of Command

Minus the stripes on the sleeve and stars on the chest, it's hard not to notice the striking similarities between the decorum and lingo of military and medical personnel. Uniforms are as ubiquitous as the orders handed down by superiors. It is easy to spot the bedraggled interns and on-call hospital residents, with stethoscopes dangling and lab coat pockets bulging with protocol notes. Attending physicians are the "generals" of the hospital, making final decisions. Resident physicians–from the chief resident down through the ranks of fourth to first year residents–are the next in command of decision makers. Each level of physician answers to the immediately higher rank of medical "officer." Similar patterns of hierarchy exist in the nursing world. The nursing staff is under the power of the physician staff and often must answer to this upper division, sometimes with disastrous consequences.

21ˢᵗ Century Tale

Susan

Susan worked nights in the ER when Jack, aged 29, came in after sustaining a head injury in a car accident. It was hard to evaluate his orientation status because Jack had been drinking heavily. The neurologist evaluated this patient and determined he should be admitted for observation but not placed in intensive care. Susan held Jack in the emergency department for a few hours so she could monitor him closely. As she observed his condition deteriorate, Susan called the neurologist at 3:00 A.M., suggesting the patient be placed under closer observation in the intensive care unit. The physician became furious at Susan's questioning of his earlier decision and refused to listen to her suggestion. Ultimately, Jack's condition did not improve overnight and he required surgery to relieve bleeding in his brain. If earlier steps had been taken, Jack might have avoided surgery, but "superior" orders superseded those of the lower ranking nurse.

It is ironic that the person for whom the hierarchy of medical care actually exists, the patient, is all too often at the bottom of the pile. Following protocols too frequently supersedes the physical, emotional, and spiritual needs of the patient.

Hierarchy is a Greek derivative from a word that means "leader of sacred rites" or "any system of persons or things ranked one above another."[36] Hierarchies are structured to delineate superior and subordinate positions. Organizational hierarchies most commonly found in medical institutions favor a structure where power and authority are held at the top with subordinates under "command"; unfortunately, subordinates seem to include patients as well as lower ranking medical staff members.

Admittedly, when managing large populations in need of acute care, whether on the battlefield or the waiting room of an urban hospital, chains of command and protocols are useful and maybe necessary-at times. The key is in discriminating between when and how to triage emergency care and considering the individual spirit and respect for a unique human life.

Triage used in acute care works. However, when the spirit is intact and the person is present—body and soul—consideration for the whole individual is essential. Typically in crisis situations, superiors bark out "orders" to get the job done. Before leaving an area, chiefs leave "Standing Orders" for the lower division workers to follow. Not following the rules exactly as written is insubordination, regardless of whether doing so is actually in the best interest of the patient. In the imbalance of an overly yang system, a hierarchical handing-down of tenets and rules breeds disrespect and disregard for the subordinates. That dynamic, in turn, breeds resentment and impinges on self-respect of the subordinates...including patients.

Given the tight reign maintained in a medical work place, tension naturally develops. Fortunately, in the last quarter century, the professional medical arena has evolved into a more friendly and cooperative work environment. However, when working in a hospital setting where life hangs in a delicate balance, the predominant western medical culture affixes blame all too quickly; that fact makes hospital work unsettling in the best of situations. Personnel, highly trained for sudden emergencies, find that their daily routine feels like walking on a high-tension wire 50 feet above the ground every moment. Most of the time the staff and physicians are not fully cognizant of this hyper-vigilance, but it is the prevailing undercurrent 24/7 inside any hospital building. Add in the constant threat of malpractice legal action and the attendant pressure of caring for each patient with perfection, and it is easy to see the burden carried by the medical institution and those who work in it. In my many years of institutional work, I noticed a lower level of compassion for each other among my co-workers. We gave great caring for our patients, significantly less caring for each other. Today the high rate of attrition of nurses is a clear indication the stressful workload this professional carries. A recent study from the University of Pennsylvania School of Nursing has found that 25 percent of practicing nurses and social workers experience "moral distress."[37] In this same study only 55.4 percent indicated that there was trust among nurses and social workers and physicians.

Fortunately, there are reports daily about small, gentle changes taking place in what seems like an inflexible system.

21st Century Tale

Gloria

Gloria recalls one particularly difficult nursing experience that was unsettling to her as a professional. She stood and watched helplessly as the already dead body of an 87-year old man named Anthony was rolled into the emergency department while his chest was violently pounded over and over again with the CPR ritual. She thought to herself, "Why can't they see that his spirit and soul are already long gone?" Without realizing she was speaking aloud, she said, "Let's just let him go in peace, not violence." Much to her surprise, the attending physician turned to her, then back to the emergency team and ordered them to halt the unnecessary protocol.

꽃

Fear, the Institutionalized Emotion

Extreme fear can neither fight nor fly.
~ William Shakespeare, The Rape of Lucrece

Fear is destructive, paralyzing. Fear is very yang; it is the opposite of yin, which is calm, flowing. Fear is opposite of the belief that "all is well," which is, after all, the goal of medical care. So, our western medical system is contradictory at the core. Here are some prevailing fears.

Fear of retribution: Staff members worry that if a proce-dure goes wrong, they might be blamed.

Fear of grief: When a patient dies, family and friends usually feel pain and loss, but occasionally they resort to anger and fault finding.

Fear of fallibility: Medical professionals expect perfec-tion from each other. If an error occurs in patient care, the guillotine descends. Many years of physician training create an aura of infallibility. The western doctor is the embodiment of the Judeo-Christian patriarch. Doctor's orders are to be followed; questioning them approaches sacrilege in a hospital. In Dr. Robert Mendelsohn's bestselling book *Confessions of a*

Medical Heretic, he names his own profession "The Church of Modern Medicine." The inside medical shenanigans he shares with the reader makes you want to run away from medical care.[38]

Fear of ego loss: The competition in pre-medical education is fierce. Top medical schools rarely consider applicants with grade averages below 3.5. Medical school has another level of competition: new physicians vie for top places in specialty residency programs such as obstetrics, orthopedics, surgical specialties, and neurosurgery. Doctors in pursuit of academic positions at prestigious colleges and universities face further competition.

Failing to achieve each of these goals, thereby missing a rung on the medical ladder, may result in a heavily bruised ego, loss of a medical specialty dream, or the reality of a lower income.

How does the competition and fear inherent in western medicine affect healing modalities? If a physician is focused on climbing the medical ladder, where are his or her thoughts at a patient's bedside? Does the patient become a victim of misplaced focus? The answers to these questions from an on-the-ground perspective reveal much inconsistency. We are all humans in this experiment called medicine. Every day, the ill are cared for, and the outcomes are often uncertain. Each person's biochemistry is different; results are rarely 100% predictable. We want to put diseases into neat categories and treat each according to a prescribed evidence-based scientific model. This mindset has tremendous limitations and strikes at the heart of the culture of malpractice legislation. A physician who does not follow the so-called "standard of care" in modern medicine, risks the loss of the license to practice. But in reality, no two people are alike; therefore, they cannot be treated exactly alike. The essence of yin medicine is to treat the individual, not the disease. Treat individually.

Anne Wilson Schaef takes this idea further. In her book *When Society Becomes An Addict*, she writes about the illusion of control in western culture. She calls it the "White Male System," or the "Addictive System." In the medical addictive system, the players are all present and accounted for: the physician plays the lead, attempting to control the helpless patient and the disease, as accompanied by the adjunct support staff, all in subordinate positions. "Our addictive system prizes control," she writes. "The Addictive System is based on fear. We fear for our very survival, and our children growing up for theirs. In a system that fosters violence and uncertainty, where confusion and self-centeredness are rampant, where the scarcity model dictates that there is often not enough food, money, time or energy (because of actual hoarding), healthy survival is a very real concern...Recovering addicts know that they must relinquish their illusion of control in order to recover. If we are to recover, we must affect a system shift."[39] The need or desire for control is based on fear. Our reliance on the western medical system is a sort of comforting addiction, where someone else holds responsibility. To recover from it requires a move from yang into a balance of yin and yang, into claiming the power and beauty of our own individual lives and our states of health.

Creative Choice, not Proscription

Just as healthy young men (and now healthy young men and women) were chosen as soldiers, medical research tended to favor these same specimens for medical research. The earliest subjects were medical students; now companies advertise for research participants, recruiting different groups of people depending on the type of research. Historically however, young (male) medical students were the "perfect" and easily accessed population. Today, pharmaceutical studies may recruit people with a certain disease, but researchers are understandably reluctant to use research pharmaceuticals on women of reproductive age who may become pregnant.

Younger males (aged 20-40) have been the popular research group for determining drug efficacy. Believe it or not, researchers did not include women as test subjects until 1992! Prior to that time, men and men alone determined drug efficacy. Imagine how a vital male (or female, for that matter) compares to a 70 or 80-year-old woman with an acute or chronic disease, slower working kidneys, and reduced circulatory capacity. These two individuals don't compare at all; their reactions to drugs don't compare, either. This older way of thinking—linear, reductionist, and once again hierarchical—has significant limitations. Scientific process, although changing in the new millennia, groups things together, classifies them as the same and then applies broad ideas and treatments. Given the uniqueness of every individual, this narrow thinking is downright deadly.

Conventional medical schools train physicians to believe that diseases are not cured but managed; patients must largely learn to live with their disease. There are two approaches for classifying disease. In the first, patients are labeled and completely identified by their disease. Doing so negates any individuality of the patient and basically obliterates hope for recovery. In the second, the disease is compartmentalized, not seen as an actual part of the patient's life and identity. This scenario is equally destructive as it gives "medicine" control over the illness and leaves the patient as a helpless pawn to be shuffled around by physicians and held hostage by high cost pharmaceuticals. NOTE: Diseases that are "cured" by surgery such as cancer are not a true cure but rather an arrest of the disease.

When an algorithm or protocol (the step-by-step management of a situation), creative thinking is left out, the patient might be lost emotionally and spiritually or even might die. Sayings such as "The operation was a success but the patient died," much like, "Winning the battle but losing the war," are all too real. Another mantra that rings too true is, "Saving lives at all cost." This military-based ideology did apply to the young men dying from battle wounds, but in general medicine it doesn't make sense in the same way. Since death is an event we will all encounter, we should honor the time of death without attaching so much fear to it. Death occurs across the full spectrum of life from infants to centenarians. When medicine operates from a one-size-fits-all mentality, everyone suffers. Patients are not identically uniformed 25-year old male victims of violence, and medical personnel are not cloned healers handing down unshakable knowledge.

Death is Part of the Process

Millions of lives have been saved due to medical leaps and bounds that came at the cost of countless other lives, many of them in battle-zone hospitals. The irony of medical progress is that much of it has come as a result of war and advancing medical technology in a time of crisis. Today in non-war situations, if we step back for a moment from the crisis scenario and just allow life to naturally flow, human health care would change. The painful lessons are clear:

quality of life is most important, especially when likely outcomes are dire. Prolonging a life just for the sake of several more days, weeks, or months in a hospital on life support is missing the point. Today in increasing numbers, people are opposed to taking "extraordinary" life saving measures. We see more and more advanced directives, living wills, and Do Not Resuscitate (DNR) requests in the medical system. Yet stories prevail where medical personnel do not honor these directives. When quality of life is lost, people lose dignity, respect, and honor. The yin respects that life flows where it wants and needs to go. Waiting and allowing the course of healing to occur honors the person; recognizing that disease is not the person is part of the respect. Yin waits and listens.

Neither the "battle" nor the "war" is lost when a person dies; the cycle of life simply continues. Regardless of varying beliefs about what happens after death, the deceased become our ancestors, worthy of honor and respect. . They are our teachers and we are the inheritors of their wisdom. Even when children die, they can become our teachers. Life is precious, and death is a part of the life cycle. The pain of death and loss are no less, but importantly we learn to accept what is; yin medicine understands this.

Connecting with the cycles of life is prevalent in many indigenous cultures; much of modern western culture emerged from earlier indigenous cultures Our ancestors understood the cycle of the seasons: The depth of winter moves forward to spring, a time of renewal and germination. Summer sees prolific growth, culminating in the summer solstice that celebrates the sun's annual zenith. The cycle continues into autumn, a time to harvest and store the bounty of gardens and fields, in preparation for the coming winter, a barren time of year. Winter is a time to go within, to hibernate, slow down, and prepare for rebirth in the next season. Staying in tune and living our lives with these cycles recognizes yin and yang time; earth and moon cycles wax and wane each month. Yang is expansion, a time of growth; yin is contraction, a time of going within to prepare for the next yang phase. In the cycle of life, both yin and yang are integral to balance. Even in a time of contraction (yin time) there is yang energy in balance. For example, on a given day I may want to be quiet, reflective and not interact with others, but I may also want to run and exercise to release pent up feelings to balance my energy.

21ˢᵗ Century Tale

Rich

Medicine was a dream of mine in high school, but the lure of a highly structured educational experience sent me in a different direction. I attended and graduated from the United States Military Academy at West Point, and served in the army as an infantry officer. I relished the fast pace of the military and the great sense of mission I felt while doing this work.

After I retired as an officer, I went on to my ultimate career: Chiropractic Medicine. I can definitely see strong similarities between the hierarchical structures of the military and medical worlds. Chiropractic medicine is so well organized in its study of anatomy, bone and muscle. But in addition to Chiropractic medicine's hard diagnoses and finite variables of form, I can still make individualized decisions, having flexibility and choice in my treatment plans. There are no overarching protocols I have to follow in my treatments as there are in the military or in a hospital. I am able to study each person, listen to who they are individually, and create a plan that works best for them.

Recently, a patient named Will came to see me, seeking help after being beaten by around his jaw, neck, and shoulders by a prisoner he was helping to incarcerate. As he came to trust me, he was able to share his difficult story with me. Listening may truly be one of the most important parts of my job now, which is entirely different from my duties in the military. Will's prognosis is very good, and he attributes much of it to being able to open up about his experiences and see healing from a more holistic prospective. Chiropractic medicine is built on the belief that the body can heal itself if it is in balance. I find that by balancing rigid structure with intuition and compassion, I have become the doctor I am today. I have the same strong sense of mission that I did when I was in the military, but now the individual rather than the algorithm dictates my approach.

Rich Hill DC, Portland, OR

❧

CHAPTER 4

Is there a Woman Doctor in the House?

∼◦๏◦∼

"I swear by Apollo Physician, by Asclepius, by Hygeia,
by Panacea and by all the gods and goddesses..."
~the first words of the Hippocratic Oath[40]

𝒜 yang viewpoint permeates the practice of medicine, with males as the predominant healthcare providers, following a militaristic model. So what about the women?

Medical Education of Women 1800-1920

In the 18th century, medical education was almost unrecognizable from what it is today. In those days, not many medical "professionals" had any formal training; gaining entrance to a school of medicine was a far less rigorous process than it is now. Men who were accepted had a connection to someone in the health care field, or enough money to afford the schools' fees. It is little surprise that before 1800, women were barred from formal education in medicine.

By the mid 1700s, no formal hospitals and only two medical schools existed in the U.S. One of those schools, King's College Medical Center New York City, founded in 1767, later became Columbia Presbyterian Medical Center. Because there were so few colleges dispensing medical knowledge, health-care education took the form of apprenticeships, as for most trades in this era.

Eighteenth century medical practitioners relied mostly on experiment and observation as the basis of their medical knowledge and treatment. Since there was no licensing or professional accreditation, and few medical schools, charlatans could practice alongside legitimate doctors. Anyone could claim healing abilities, establish a practice, and charge to treat patients. And many people did! These phonies might be driven out of town for their false practices, only to set up in a new location. Eventually, public reaction against the quacks helped to establish a more organized system of medical training and delivery.

As America grew from the early 1800s on, medical colleges sprung up and expanded. These first schools followed an apprenticeship format, where students worked closely with a mentor. Soon, medical schools proliferated in such rapid numbers that the quality of education was compromised. From 1810 to 1840, 26 new medical schools opened. From 1840 until about 1910, 46 new schools were established. Few of these schools were associated with hospitals. Instead, they were privately owned, designed as moneymaking business ventures. The emphasis on profit reduced the educational quality of these schools. No entrance exams were required and no exit exams tested a graduate's proficiency. Quite simply, if you were male and had the means to pay for this training you were, voila, a doctor.

Female Impact on Medicine

Finally, in 1850, the state of Pennsylvania passed a law that permitted women's education in medicine, paving the way for medical schools to admit women. Just three years earlier, in 1847, Geneva Medical College in New York reluctantly admitted Elizabeth Blackwell to its school, after she received repeated rejections from colleges in both New York and Philadelphia.[41] When she graduated in 1849, she became the first woman in America to earn a medical degree, and she did so with the highest grades in her class. This courageous, intelligent, and compassionate woman had a huge impact on medical care for women and children. Because she had so often heard complaints from women who preferred to be treated by a doctor of their own sex, she took action. Dr Blackwell and her sister, Emily Blackwell, opened the New York Infirmary for Women and in 1857, a medical school, the Women's Medical College.[42] She was also the author of several important textbooks on women's medicine.

Later, she taught gynecology and hygiene in New York and London hospitals, and formed the National Health Society in the United Kingdom. But Dr. Blackwell's impact reached even further. At her college, she raised the standard of medical training by insisting on stricter admission and graduation requirements. Students took entrance exams, studied for longer periods of time, and were tested by examining boards upon completion of their training. No other medical school of the time imposed these requirements. Her feats are all the more amazing because she accomplished them beneath the harsh criticism of unfriendly male colleagues. Dr. Blackwell's contributions to medicine were far-reaching and had a tremendous impact on its practice.

Dr. Blackwell's establishment of a women's college began to change the prevailing thought about the competence and intellect of women. At the time, men fiercely opposed women receiving any higher education. Male physicians also paid less attention to poorer populations. As a result, health care for women and children suffered, with the poorer among them receiving little to no medical care.

Even a luminary such as Florence Nightingale was initially against women becoming physicians. She felt that women could serve other women best by becoming nurses or midwives, and focusing on diseases that affected women and children. To Nightingale, a nursing education was far superior to a medical school education because the latter required rote memorization. By contrast, nurses' training at the time was much more practical and useful. She stated, "Medical education is about as bad as it possibly can be. It makes men arrogant (prigs). It prevents any wise, any philo-sophical, any practical view of health and disease. Only a few geniuses rise above it."[43]

Years later, Nightingale did change her stance on the education of women as physicians, after significant mile-stones were made educating women in England. Her motto on women's opportunity for medical education became, "Give us free trade and let the public decide."[44]

Another healing modality emerged during the mid 1800s, and its primary adherents were women. This practice was called hydropathy and utilized water therapy to cure disease. Women, perhaps drawn to it by its gentle nature, wholeheartedly embraced this practice. (Note: To avoid confu-sion between hydrotherapy vs. hydropathy, hydropathy is the use of quantities of water – both internally and externally – to treat pathology or disease. Hydrotherapy is the external use of water as the main healing component, often in temperature contrasts.[45])

The "Hydropathy Movement" was greatly criticized and scorned by the AMA's medical lobby. The movement lost favor with allopaths in the last part of the 19th century in this power struggle. The striking irony is that hygienists practiced with water and focused on prevention more than disease, but ended up losing ground when the AMA formed the Department of Health in 1898.[46] Hygienists were excluded from this new government organization.

The practice of hydropathy began in Europe and moved across the Atlantic. Introduced in New York State, it took root and flourished in many parts of America. Because hydropathy was a gentle and non-invasive practice, it quickly gained a following. Water cure doctors proliferated in the New England and the Mid-Atlantic states, as well as in the Ohio River Valley, where sanitariums sprouted up. Eventually hydropathy moved as far west as Oregon and California.

Hydropathy as a system of medicine encouraged women to become strong and self-reliant, promoting self-care and disease prevention. This was quite a change from the predominant view of women at the time as fragile, helpless, and prone to fainting. The therapy grew due to the hard work, determination, and dedication of the many female hydropathy practitioners. In the sanitariums where the therapy was practiced, women could board and enjoy the pleasures of a simple diet, fresh air, rest, recreation, and socialization, as well as the water therapies. The treatments were less caustic than other medical practices; further, women could learn to duplicate treatments for themselves and their children at home.

This aspect of the therapy appealed to women, the traditional guardians of their family's health. Women of the era enjoyed water therapy's emphasis on self-reliance and the curative powers of nature. It also provided women with a viable alternative for dealing with health problems at a time when orthodox therapies frequently were dangerous, distasteful, and ineffective.[47] The predominant paradigm at the time was "Heroic Medicine," a model which lasted approximately from 1780 to 1850.

Heroic Medicine describes the standard medical procedures of the time, which included the use of aggressive tactics and harsh medicines, such as emetics and cathartics, to treat diseases. Doctors used bloodletting and sweating, as well as calomel, a mercury compound, to make patients regurgitate and rid their bodies of impurities. Death from these therapies often was worse than the disease itself.[48]

So it is no surprise that women embraced the far gentler use of water therapy in place of these harsh treatments. In *Wash and Be Healed*, author Susan Cayleff notes the popularity of water douches, sitz baths, and thermal and herbal baths. Hydropathy offered an innovative approach to easing pregnancy, childbirth, and the postpartum period.

Water cure adherents maintained a feminist perspective on health care, particularly concerning a woman's clothing. Hydropathic reformers encouraged women to abandon such fashionable but constricting and health-impairing clothing as the corset. They also urged females to acquire anatomical and physiological knowledge of their bodies.

The hydropathic profession was a boon to women's rights and female health-care practitioners because it actively recruited and supported women as physicians and health lecturers. Water therapists urged women to help themselves through the study of medicine, and thus the hydropathic movement was intertwined with the rise of female physicians.

Women owned many of the water healing centers that existed during this time, and they in turn hired female practitioners, preferred by their predominantly female clientele. Largely through the influence of hydrotherapy, this was an encouraging time for women.

One of the leading pioneers in hydrotherapy was Mary Gove Nichols (1810-1884), who launched the movement in America and, combining the principles of water-cure therapy with health reform, became a role model to women. Nichols believed that when women gained control of their physiological health they also gained control of their futures.

Her husband, Thomas Nichols MD, and she started a hydrotherapy school and opened popular sanitariums that offered the gentle therapies of rest, natural foods, and often mineral water treatment. The duo also opened a variety of clinics and institutes dedicated to better health, and both were prolific writers who were widely published in the water journals of the day.[49] The *Water Cure Journal* was the most popular of regularly-published periodicals read by the general population especially lay women followers. Many practitioners, including women authors, contributed to this journal.[50]

However, despite the rise of women as health-care workers, and the strides being made in women's health, the number of women trained as physicians still remained small; men's domination of the medical profession continued to grow.

Women and Birthing

Prior to the Civil War (1861-1865), complications of and death from childbirth and the postpartum phase caused the early deaths of many women. Childbed or puerperal fever ran rampant in institutional settings. Post partum infection was a serious, life-threatening disease resulting in a significant number of maternal deaths. The use of calomel and blood-letting were the standard treatments for postpartum sepsis (an overwhelming systemic infection). While statistics are unavailable from this time, it was common knowledge that poor women attended by female midwives did not suffer as greatly as, and had fewer complications than, well-to-do women attended by male medical personnel.

However, this era also saw the rise of the "new" obstetrics, which spread from the United Kingdom. Male midwives, who practiced among urban middle- and upper-class women, moved this field of medicine away from its traditional arena as a woman's healing art. Through time, it became a legitimate branch of male-controlled medicine.

Alarmingly, the number of cases of puerperal fever rose with the growth of male-midwifery. Though some male doctors began to suspect that the fever was contagious and its spread linked to poor hygiene, others ridiculed the notion. As early as the 1770's, British surgeon Charles White hypothesized a relationship between puerperal fever, retention of a woman's bodily fluids (lochia), and infection. He urged physicians to wash women with mild astringents and have the women sit up after childbirth. Oliver Wendell Holmes, Sr., also recognized the connection when a surgeon friend contracted puerperal fever after dissecting the body of an infected woman. Thus, he reasoned, physicians were directly responsible for the fever's transmission.

In earlier centuries, statistics about women's childbearing were not kept. However, it was common knowledge that births attended by women had fewer complications and deaths than those attended by men. This was finally confirmed in records kept by Dr. Charles White in 1772.[51]

At the same time in Vienna, Dr. Ignaz Semmelweis stressed the need to observe strict hygienic routines for women's lying-in rooms. He insisted on hand washing between working on autopsies and examining birthing mothers, which made him a laughing stock among his peers. American obstetricians also denied that puerperal fever was contagious, and it would be another twenty years before hand washing became an acceptable and subsequently standard medical practice.[52]

However, many women without formal training who assisted in the birth process did so without inflicting the complication of puerperal fever on their patients, simply by washing their hands and using water in birthing. Bathing and comforting those in their care was a natural expression of the maternal instinct in female birthing assistants. Thus, women who were delivered by medical doctors had three times higher rates of puerperal fever than those who were delivered by female midwives.[53] Authors Richard and Dorothy Wertz are perplexed why this country has made a natural process such as birth into a medical one. "We strongly suspect that such extensive and regular medicalization was unnecessary, was often dangerous and dehumanizing, and was primarily the product of a long-term, relentless and pervasive effort by doctors to control birth, to technologize, institutionalize, and ultimately denaturalize and standardize it. "[54]

Female midwives have felt strongly that childbirth was a natural event and not something relegated to institutions for the sick and dying. Admittedly, some advances in obstetrics had been a boon for women, but for the most part the medicalization of childbirth was and is a detriment to the birthing mother. Now, in the 21st century, we witness a strong movement back to home births and birthing centers separate from hospitals. As women take back their bodies, more births take place at home or home-like birth centers just as it took place before the popularity of institutions.

Since the 1960s, the process of giving birth has improved. However, not that long ago, women were still shackled to the delivery room table. As an example of some of the horrors of those days, here is my own personal birth story of my first born.

"Sorry, your husband can't come along with you," the admitting clerk of the hospital said.

"But why can't he?" I asked.

"It's against hospital rules," she replied.

And so I kissed my husband goodbye, as another contraction caused me to arch my back and I was whisked away to the labor and delivery department. As an RN at the suburban hospital where I was about to deliver this baby, you would have thought I'd have known that my husband wouldn't be with me. But I didn't. Nor did I have any idea what to expect over the next six hours of laboring, which would culminate in the birth of our first-born son.

I didn't have any personal experience of labor, except to witness, during my nurse's training, the poor Hispanic women of Manhattan's lower east side deliver their babies. The obstetrical department in that big city hospital was a baby mill, and it did not inspire me to specialize in obstetrical nursing. Too often I witnessed this group of women treated without respect during this most sacred event. I had some concerns, too about the lack of deep caring during this intimate and momentous occasion. Procedures that had to be followed and protocols that must be met were more important than the human element.

In my hospital labor room, I endured the humiliation

of the routine pubic shave and enema; then, the contractions occupied my entire attention. They were coming hard, strong, and long, and I quickly shed my earlier modesty about who saw me or what body part they viewed. Alone in my room, I writhed back and forth on the steel-railed bed, afraid to yell out in pain. Some relief came when I received a narcotics injection to supposedly help me "sleep" between contractions.

"How long does this go on?" I asked the empty room. It didn't answer. And I had no answers, either, despite the fact that I was a nurse and should have known what to expect. But I didn't. I had no clue.

Parts of this story are difficult to write, revealing as they are about a profession I love so much. Nursing was my passion. Yet here I was, in terrible pain, all alone. I could not understand why I had been brought here without my husband. *Be brave and don't let others know you feel, I thought.* Hours passed rather quickly with my drugged mind. More relief came when they injected another drug into my back. As I became unable to move anything from my waist down, my feeling of helplessness grew.

Soon I heard a voice say, "Yup, she's ready. Bring her in here."

At last I was having this baby!

What took place in the next hour almost seems unbelievable, although it was routine in most delivery rooms in the 1960s. I was lifted onto a table as my legs still could not operate on their own, and then I was strapped into padded metal gridirons that forced me into a wide split. I felt the pull in my groin but I did not realize that my hip joints could move in those directions. At this point the spinal anesthetic given to relieve the pain of contractions began to wear off.

"The head is crowning!" I heard someone say.

I was excited. It was finally happening! I asked that mirrors be placed so that I could witness this momentous event myself. But when I attempted to raise myself up so that I could see, I felt leather straps on my arms. I was restrained! The next voice I heard told me to breathe deeply. A mask with anesthesia was put on my face ....I was gone. Gone from this beautiful event. Robbed of the exhilaration of my son's emergence. The next thing I realized, my baby was lying on my stomach; as I reached out to stroke him, the wrist restraints again held me back. I lowered my head, defeated.

So much in these last few minutes was lost:

I lost my husband's support and caring

I lost the view of my child's birth.

I lost my chance to stroke and touch him and welcome him into the world.

This was the medical world that I was a part of. And, at the time, my 22-year-old mind had no words for it.

Women Gain, then Lose Status

In the last half of the 19th century, the 155 medical schools in the US were largely unregulated. In an effort to make medical education universal and to improve the training of doctors, industrialist Andrew Carnegie hired and funded Abraham Flexner to visit each medical school in America, examining the schools' training programs and laboratory facilities. In 1910, the Flexner Report, supported by the AMA, was published with a goal to set new standards for the practice of medicine. This report spelled doom for women's medical colleges, homeopathic colleges, and southern black colleges, closing most of them within the next decade.[55]

Why? The problem lay with advances in laboratory

science, which were enthusiastically embraced by medical authorities. They considered only strict adherence to current scientific principles as acceptable; any eclectic or wisdom-based medical care was considered unscientific and unsafe. Many of these same attitudes prevail today. Because the bulk of women's colleges were poorly funded, they lacked the supposedly requisite laboratory facilities or a hospital affiliation. However, in these schools, the focus of healing was simply different. They sought to bring medical care to the poor who could not afford the expensive white male doctors.

Yet, because of the Flexner Report, the women's, homeopathic, and black medical colleges were closed. No more would women treat women; no more would black communities have medical practitioners who understood their unique medical needs (some of which were the results of slavery).

At first after the closure of the women's colleges, women remained confident that co-educational medical programs would expand. However, the Flexner Report succeeded in closing all but three of the 155 medical colleges in existence.[56] The three remaining medical schools accepted only elite, educated ,white males; women were edged out of the admissions pool. A commonly held belief at the time was that a woman's delicacy and her monthly cycle made her unsuitable for the noble medical profession. What was the result of these events? Medical doctors enjoyed an exclusive market because suddenly there were many fewer trained physicians. Because these physicians could regulate standard practices and fees, a medical monopoly was born.

Some critics have called this the medical cartel of elitism. Harvard medical school was one of the three surviving schools, but it ceased admitting women until 1946.[57] This was especially ironic, given that America's first female physician, Dr. Elizabeth Blackwell, along with her sister Emily, helped raise money to keep the doors of Harvard open.

Despite all these barriers, and the continuing criticism they faced for learning about the human body, women continued to seek medical educations. Many discovered that nursing, midwifery, and the ministry were friendlier avenues for females and sought training in those disciplines. Others used a different approach.

Dr. Maria Zakrezewska founded the New England Hospital for Women and Children, located in Boston. She wrote to Dr. Blackwell about her practice of medicine and held the belief that women physicians had to out shine their male counterparts. She also noted her preference for teaching her patients preventative hygiene also serving the poor populations by teaching sanitation, nutrition, hygiene, and ventilation.[58] At the same time, Dr. Blackwell is noted for saying that women are needed in the medical profession for their "spiritual power of maternity."[59]

Why were women kept from practicing medicine? This is a complex question with answers not only in the trends just mentioned, but also in the social Victorian climate that dominated formal scientific and medical training in the 19th century. The prevailing view of women's place as a secondary citizen was strong.

Whether a woman could rise above that dominance depended on the cultural milieu in which she lived. In America and Europe, she simply was unable to rise above male dominance in politics and education.

As Mary Putnam Jacobi, the first woman to become a member of the American Academy of Medicine and a fierce proponent of educational opportunities for women, wrote

married Benedict Lust, a famous nature cure physician who studied with Father Sebastian Kneipp in Austria and brought the water cure to America. Louisa owned and operated a popular sanitarium in Butler, New Jersey, where she taught the importance of a healthful environment and good nutrition. Dr. Lust was admired for her simple and straightforward nature cure methods, which she shared with all her clients. With her deep knowledge of nutrition and dietetics, she prepared meals for the sanitarium residents and in 1907 published her book, *The Practical Naturopathic Vegetarian Cook Book.* Reprints of this book are still available today.[62] When she died at age 57, the profession of naturopathy lost an important figure. Louisa Lust provided unending support for Benedict, her husband. She was the financial as well as moral support for her husband's campaign to promote and establish water cure medicine in the New York area. The authors of *The Nature Doctors* comment. "The naturopathic profession owes an unacknowledged debt to Louisa Lust. Throughout this century, thousands of naturopaths, unaware of the influence she wielded, have been able to practice naturopathic medicine because of her efforts."[63]

Undaunted Women

In 1894, only 10% of the medical student population was female.[64] By the end of the 19th century, pioneering women had established nineteen women's colleges and nine women's hospitals all across America. The number of American physicians was 7,000, of which still only 4-5% were women.[65] Over the span of 120 years (1850 – 1970), the status of women in medicine changed only by small degrees. Small numbers of women earned degrees to practice medicine, while the number of male medical practitioners grew more quickly. In some urban areas, female medical school graduates were restricted or barred from opportunities for a residency position. Undaunted, women flourished in rural settings wherever a doctor was needed. Stories abound of women who conducted medical clinics from their kitchens, indigenous cultural centers, workplaces, and industrial depots. Women donated unending hours of service to their communities. And yet, American law still restricted women from having their full voice. Women could not vote or serve on juries until 1920.

Few women entered politics, and few to no women held CEO positions. We must honor these women, and remember not only the odds they faced, but also the endless courage it took to pursue a career they were well suited for and yet often denied. It is well recognized today that women are natural doctors, but these women of history moved far beyond the stereotypical female; they maintained focus on their innate qualities to love and serve others. This was, and still is, women's medicine.

21ˢᵗ Century Tale

Deborah

At 5' 2," Deborah Francis is a naturopathic doctor who stands tall and looks people directly in their eyes as she speaks her truth of healing ways. A healer and spiritual teacher, she says she is done tiptoeing around the medical establishment and now speaks about the herbal spirits that resonate with her. Her shamanic initiation moved her away from her career as a psychiatric RN for more than 10 years. Her spirit guides led her to naturopathic medicine. People love to hear her insights into the spirit of medicinal plants: she talks to them and they share their valuable healing secrets. She is well trained in the sciences, yet she walks closely on the earth communicating with plants.

Although part Native American, she was unaware of her heritage until fifteen years ago. She says, however, that something inside her always knew. She recalls a memory from her early childhood when she wanted to know how to use plants and how to communicate with animals. "I loved being out in nature—it just felt so right for me." She gained a sense of relief upon learning of her Lakota tribe ancestry, finally knowing where she really belonged.

As a psychiatric nurse, she worked with heavily-medicated patients whom she recognized as very sensitive people. "They hated being on the drugs," she remembers, "and I hated giving them out." She moved away from psychiatry to work as an intensive care unit (ICU) nurse. "It broke my heart to see the devastating effects drugs had on people. The most disturbing case was a 35-year-old asthmatic woman who suffered from osteoporosis, which caused fractures in her upper spine (thoracic vertebrae). The disease arose over the years from the drugs she had taken for her asthma. She still could not breathe well and now had unrelenting pain from the fractures." This kind of experience inspired Deborah to leave her nursing career, declaring there had to be something better.

That better place is using gentler medicine, taking time with each patient, and inviting the spirits for healing help.

❧

CHAPTER 5

Healing Does Matter

~⟨℮⟩~

Intuition is the root of most scientific breakthroughs.
~ Barbara Braham

At the very dawn of humankind, the human female was
regarded as a prodigious source of wisdom and power.
She could bring life and save life, and therefore was the healer
of sick bodies and wandering souls.
~ Jeanne Achterberg

While woman's innate wisdom has been alive and well for all the millennia since human life first began, recognition of it, and its attendant social status, has waxed and waned. At times her wisdom was lauded; at others, she kept it secret.

Recovery of Her Healing Power

Early recorded history indicates that woman and all that her femininity symbolized were adored. She was greatly honored both for her reproductive abilities, but also because she ruled the home. The tribe depended on her not only for the growth of the clan but also for its survival. Man was the hunter who provided food, but woman was head of the tribe and made the critical decisions.[66] Many recent archaeological discoveries in ancient burial sites substantiate female position and power from these earliest times, showing there was considerably less warfare or fighting before

2,000 BC.[67] Man did not emerge as a warrior until later.

But slowly, very slowly over time, woman's status eroded and changed. Fighting over land, power, and relationships ensued. Soon, the male sword became more powerful than the female heart. Men triumphed and overpowered women's position not only in the family, but also in the clans and tribes. Men moved about the continent, taking control through killing and enslaving others, often mostly women.[68]

Woman's knowledge and ownership of her wisdom are beginning to resurface and take their rightful place in history. What would the evolution of medicine have been like if women's education was equal to men's? I posit that today's medicine would have a very different presentation to the patient: feelings of warmth and caring would predominate. Healing and a standard of care incorporating equal parts of yin and yang principles would be the norm of medical care. It is clear that women affect changes in healing.

The Role of Women Healers

Women, by virtue of their unique biology, have an innate urge to nurture others. The process of female reproduction, with its influx of hormones during pregnancy and childbirth, bathes the brain in bio-chemicals that awaken the instinct to care for family.[69] And when I say "family," I refer also to the extended families that often exist in rural towns and villages. Early archaeological findings reveal that women cared for the whole family by preparing and providing food that assured survival. Men were often gone from the homestead, hunting or doing other work.

In her role as the center of the family, a woman also, by necessity, learned how to nurse her family when they fell ill. Women shared effective remedies with other women; in this way they learned from each other. Most healing traditions found in indigenous cultures were passed on by word of mouth, not written down. Most ancient cultures had oral traditions in every aspect of their lives; the lack of a written language does not render oral wisdom less valuable.

A great number of today's pharmaceutical products have their origins in plants; plant medicine was, and still is, the essence of how women throughout the world care for themselves. One example of a well-used pharmaceutical is the medicine digitalis. The origin of this drug is the foxglove, which produces a beautiful flower. Foxglove is a deadly herb if not used correctly, but in very small doses, it can be a lifesaver for a failing heart. Centuries ago, an English herbalist discovered foxglove's properties and physician William Withering documented its use. However, female herbalists have used plants as medicine for thousands of years. As Jeanne Achterberg notes, "A tea of foxglove leaves had been used by the wise women for centuries. It was only when Dr. Withering's fiancée persuaded him to visit an old woman herbalist that he became aware of the plant's medicinal properties."[70] Too often women's innate knowledge has been sidelined by so-called scientific data, omitting credit where credit is due.

Another example supporting the importance of women's work and ideas comes from the smallpox epidemic of 1872 in England[71,72]. Edward Jenner is credited with developing the smallpox vaccination that eventually eradicated the disease. However, once again women had known that inoculation was helpful in disease for millennia. As Achterberg says, "European wise women also had been performing similar injections (vaccinations) probably for centuries prior to the 1700's."[73]

The wise woman prepared her plant medicines in the kitchen, along with her family's food. This room was the center of the home, where all essential activities took place, since it contained the hearth and, later, the stove. The kitchen was also where people bathed, where women applied healing poultices or cleaned wounds. The kitchen was woman's domain. From here, she orchestrated household activities and cared for others in time of need. The woman of the house was the natural go-to person in times of crisis and care. She was the center.

Outside her kitchen women's power did not remain. Women had little option but to stay home, busy raising, caring for, and feeding large families. Women did form small groups to self educate, but gradually they became more removed from centers of higher education and their advantage was lost.

Today, as the world shrinks due to global trade and internet communications, knowledge and power are becoming more equal. The common perception throughout history and today is that men's knowledge is superior to women's. However, it is my belief that women's knowledge was and is essential for the continuation and preserving life. Yet woman lost her equality long ago and she still has not fully regained it.

Who Turned the Tide?

Earlier chapters discussed women such as Hildegarde of Bingen, Trotula of Salerno, Florence Nightingale, and Dr. Elizabeth Blackwell. Each of these women contributed outstanding work to their fields. And yet, none of them had the momentum to step into their fullest power and lead women out of the oppressive cultural norms of the time. However, since 1990, thanks to the strong leadership of a few brave women, the tide is at least turning. And as women rise into higher and higher decision-making positions, the status of women will continue to evolve.

Bernadine Healy, MD, is an outstanding example of a woman making a significant medical decision that changed history. As director of the National Institute for Health (NIH), a major research institute, she mandated that no further studies could be done on men alone, if the disease being studied also affected women. This seems so obvious, but before Dr. Healy, medical researchers only studied men. The long-term practice in science has been to conduct most research on males, both human and animal, but not on females. Women's estrous, or menstrual, cycle increased the challenge of conducting consistent studies with women subjects. Or so the researchers claimed. To their credit scientific researchers wanted to avoid potentially harming or interfering with a pregnancy. But the push for reliable data, coupled with the challenge of studying women, meant that ultimately male scientists ignored them. Yet now we know the absence of studies specifically focused on women has resulted in biased data, data that does not apply to women, but that scientists use to define conditions and prescribe treatment.

Because of Healy's influence, a whole new specialty arose: Women's Medicine.

Dr. Healy made a significant impact in this arena, vastly changing women's medical treatment by burning a hole through years of indifference to women's medical needs. A graduate of Harvard Medical School with top honors, Healy went on to complete her cardiology residency at Johns Hopkins School of Medicine. Since then, she has enjoyed a stellar career, attaining a full professorship at Johns Hopkins and appointed the first woman to head up the National Institute for Health (NIH), where she directed and oversaw notable studies on women's cardiovascular health. Under her leadership, the NIH launched the $625 million Women's Health Initiative, a long-term health study involving 150,000 women.[74]

When asked about her accomplishments, Dr. Healy said, "My contributions on women's health and well-being including the Women's Health Initiative, which I envisioned and launched while at the National Institutes of Health, have brought me deep satisfaction—and were not always easy...."[75].

This important paradigm shift deserves a closer look, examining how women innately resonate with yin energy.

The Essence of Healing - Nurturance

The basic definition of nurturance is providing care and attention. The role woman has traditionally played in raising her children and caring for her family and community is of focused, kind attention and care. She has had millions of years to practice nurturing, because it has always been her primary role. The traditional and opposite male role is that of doer, fixer and provider. Both roles are important for human survival, and both deserve honor for what they've accomplished. However, in the practice of modern medicine, the cry of the wounded from the battlefield still echoes and the warrior paradigm remains the dominant method of treating the sick and injured. Yang medicine. When yin medicine, with its welcoming precepts, is invited in, the healing and curing journey can be very different.

Touch

The power of touch is vital to the process of healing. For humans to grow they need food and shelter. Yet touch is also required for them to thrive. Studies show that babies will not thrive and often die when they are not touched, held, and nurtured in the early infant years. In a study reported in the *Early Childhood Education Journal*, pre-term infants massaged fifteen minutes three times a day for ten days gained 47% more weight and stayed in the hospital for a shorter time than infants who did not receive consistent touch during the study.[76]

Touch is a basic human need. Touching skin surfaces has soothing and relaxing qualities. In the past 30 to 40 years, courageous and intuitive women healers have re-established touch as a healing modality. One of these is Dolores Krieger, RN, PhD, a pioneer in the realm of Therapeutic Touch (TT); her work demonstrates yin medicine. A nursing professor emerita, Krieger taught at New York University in the 1970s and popularized her method through the university's advanced nursing program.[77] She also took TT beyond the campus to a worldwide stage, and subsequently many people have trained in her TT method throughout the world. Dora Kunz, the originator of TT and a collaborator of Dr. Krieger's, states, "Therapeutic Touch is a universal healing energy available to all living beings."[78] Krieger and Kunz validated what mothers, fathers, and healers of all cultures instinctively know: touch that is loving and caring is life nurturing. TT methods help alleviate pain, speed healing of surgical wounds, and create a sense of peace within both the healer and the one being healed. Based on her years of research, Krieger's has documented these results, as well as those of premature babies flourishing with the TT method.[79]

And yet, the scientific world has conveyed mixed messages about the value of touch. There are detractors who denounce the scientific effects of hands-on healing. What is true, whether proven by science or not, is that touching another human with positive intent heals by its comforting, soothing effects, and from a basic energetic connection.[80]

Another form of healing touch is shiatsu. This ancient method of healing touch has a rich and long cultural history, dating before the practice of acupuncture. In shiatsu, practitioners use their fingers to apply pressure to precise points on the body, specifically for healing.[81] Interestingly, some of the earliest shiatsu healers were blind. Waichi Sugiyama (1614-1694) eliminated the severe abdominal pain that a Japanese master shogun (a military commander) suffered after his physicians had been unable to help him. The successful shiatsu treatment eventually led to the establishment of Shiatsu schools and training for blind people in this art.[82]

Woman's work in her family brings her in touch with her children as well as the sick or injured whom she nurses. She touches them as she bathes them and applies lotions, liniments, or other soothing salves. She holds babies and children in their growing years. She wraps and tucks them into bed, as a sign of warmth and caring. This is woman's work, and it is healing.

Another example of touch is the work of Laura Peterson. Her organization is called *Hands to Hearts International* a relatively new grass-roots movement. Peterson felt the call to help impoverished people of the world and subsequently founded her organization. Laura's vision is to teach women and men the importance of connecting to their young children in the first three to five years of life. The goal is to help them make a difference in their world, rising out of the poverty that entraps them.

Volunteers go into villages and help parents, mostly mothers, in holding the little ones and singing and playing with them. This work is transforming individual lives and whole communities. It is a perfect example of the power of one woman's vision embracing the yin – love, connection, and touch. To quote Peterson's website, "Researchers and policy makers around the world are understanding that early childhood is the most effective time to improve a person's life."[83]

Music

Music heals. Music is universal. Music can touch you like a prayer.

Research has shown that the use of songs, chants, prayers, spells, and music produce emotional states in a patient that affect the way the immune system responds to illness.[84] Vibration, rhythm, and sound appear universally in cultures. In many indigenous cultures, the shaman heals with ceremonial performances that use dance and song. The rhythm of the drum resonates with the human vibration. Shamans often talk of their work as coming from a dream state or "other" world. When the shaman moves the person being healed into this altered state, worldly stresses disappear and endorphin levels rise. Endorphins, the natural bio-chemicals of the brain, aid healing by supporting the immune system,[85] and can reduce the pain and anxiety often associated with illness.

The origins of music likely trace back to the sounds of nature and to chanting in spiritual realms. Indigenous people even today understand the uplifting and connecting effects of music and chanting. According to Mitchell Gaynor, modern music therapy is likely an outgrowth of the shamanic sound healing of 30,000 years ago.[86] Music therapy today is used in many types of healing for its variety of vibration patterns: some patterns calm and soothe the senses; others stimulate the person to a joyous level. Most music can create a positive experience for the listener.

Music is useful in a variety of ways in both healing and home care settings. Music calms those making their transition in death. Elders with Alzheimer's disease and other dementias, as well as autistic children, respond to music's rhythmic sounds and familiar patterns. And mothers of diverse cultures sing or hum to their babies to calm them.

Studies that measure the physiologic effects of music on body functions show results such as lowered blood pressure, heart rate and cortisol levels (Cortisol is a stress hormone.) and increased immune cell activity. Another reported result of music therapy is raised endorphin levels, which have an opiate effect on the patient.[87]

Music has a universal appeal: people of all ages, in most cultures throughout time, relish rhythmic sounds and music. The author of *Sounds of Healing*, Mitchell Gaynor, notes, "I see the interplay and balance required to make music as a reflecltion of the harmonious interaction of the nervous, endocrine, and immune systems in a health body."[88]

Words and States of Mind

The words we say to ourselves–and to others–have an effect on our health and well-being. Today many spiritual teachings, including New Thought, Science of Mind, and Buddhism, teach the power of thoughts and words. Evangelical speakers such as Billy Graham and peace-loving individuals such as Nelson Mandela and Mother Theresa have shown the world that much is accomplished by the power of positive words. In the 1940's and 1950's, Norman Vincent

Peale articulated the power of positive thinking. One of his famous quotes is, "Change your thoughts and you change your world."

We are what we think and say; that is the message of the wildly popular book, *The Secret*, by Rhonda Byrnes. This message is echoed in medical lore. Physicians who give a patient a specific timeline to live with a terminal disease are never surprised when the patient dies right on schedule. Those who live beyond the predictions for themselves are the ones who fill themselves with positive thoughts and a positive outlook. They very often get a positive outcome by living longer!

Words in the form of affirmations heal the mind. The words we think and speak direct our lives. Thus, people use affirmations to bring good into their lives. And conversely, negative thinking and speaking can affect our physical bodies. Douglas Bloch writes that through repetition of a word or phrase, you create a magnetic field that attracts the desired condition to you. He states: "Thought is magnetic. In life, we receive what we attract. And what we attract is determined by our most deeply held beliefs."[89]

Many writers, philosophers, and spiritual teachers have documented the benefit of both positive words and time spent in quiet moments. Women, too, have known this for centuries, singing sweet words to their children to reassure them when frightened, or simply to give them a positive outlook. These techniques result in an improved state of mind for adults and children alike.

Further, it is well documented that a meditative state produces distinct and positive physiological changes.[90] Time spent sitting quietly, without words, in a state of relaxation, has great healing effects. Words of prayer, too, can create healing. Larry Dossey, MD, writes about the power of prayer in healing but is frank in his opening comments, saying that medical professionals and scientists are "poorly informed about the empirical evidence surrounding prayer."[91]

Whether you do or do not believe in prayer, changing our frame of mind can be a tremendous healer. Change can come by emptying or clearing the mind, changing the thoughts or releasing old ideas and beliefs. This is an aspect of medicine that often stays outside the conversation about illness, but could be included in discussions with your doctor or health care provider.

Water

Water is one of the most useful and powerful liquids on earth; it sustains life. We are completely bathed in water for the first nine months of our life inside the womb. Our bodies are more than 70% water, which regulates the body's physiology. And water is, of course, yin. It flows, and it is interchangeable from solid (ice), to liquid, to gas (steam). Water is the carrier of nutrients, so it helps to feed us. It also regulates our body temperature. We can fast from food for weeks or months, but we cannot live without water for more than a few days.

Yin medicine is closely associated with water, because of its grounding, nurturing, dark, and deep properties. Water is soothing, caressing, and calming. Walk along a river, stream, ocean, or gentle waterfall, and you'll soon feel calmness come over you, due to the negative ions created by moving water. Even taking a shower creates negative ions! These particles are healers because they neutralize free radicals, which cause cell damage in our bodies. This is one reason why we tend to feel good around water.

Healers know this intuitively. Both trained and untrained healers have practiced water therapies for millennia. Hot water therapies bring warmth and ease, while cold-water therapies stimulate and increase tonicity. Tepid water (96 to 98 degrees) reduces anxiety, induces relaxation, and helps calm hyperactive states. Before psychiatric drugs were available, neutral baths were a common effective treatment. Planet earth provides many types of geothermal mineral waters with springs all over the globe. Since recorded time, people have soaked, bathed and healed in the "waters." Native Americans utilized these powerful waters in both ceremony and for health. When settlers came to this continent, they learned about these hot water sources from the native people. By the nineteenth century a number of these geothermal springs became healing centers attracting people far and wide to " take the waters." Their popularity grew into the twentieth century, but lost favor when the pharmaceutical market developed and captured people's attention with a quick "cure." Fast acting post World War II medicine was emerging. Some well known centers were Saratoga Hot Springs in New York, Hot Springs of Arkansas, Calistoga Hot Springs in California. Revival in the hot mineral springs tradition is growing again, but many of the earlier places have fell into great disrepair. Still the interest remains for people who understand the value to earth's water gift – her yin gift.

The work women do often utilizes water including bathing loved ones and the sick. Traditionally women perform a ritual bath for the body of those who have just died. As a young nurse it was one of the most solemn and respectful rituals I was taught in nursing; I bathed my first deceased patient as a nineteen-year-old student. Childbirth, for much of history, used water, with some propounding the benefits of underwater births. Preparing and cooking food, another traditional woman's domain, requires water. Cleanliness, both personal and for the surrounding environment, is also a woman's art, and it requires water.

The healing qualities of yin are not exclusive to women; some males who also participate in these practices. Benedict Lust, ND, campaigned long and hard to establish water therapies in America; others joined him in his crusade. The continuing problem is that the scientific community does not readily welcome yin modalities. When introduced, these modalities were at first scoffed at and then relegated to a back seat, seen as second rate or quackery. We may be finally coming back full circle.

21st Century Tale

Babs

My mother was a nurse, so as a young woman I thought of myself in that role. I always knew I wanted to help people but did not know what helping people would look like. Nursing seemed like the place to find out. My inspiration came when working as a nurse's aide, watching the staff of nurses give deeply nurturing, tender care to a young man with a spinal cord injury. I also remember a burn patient who was nurtured in a warm, thoughtful way. It touched me.

While studying in my nursing program I also took night classes in what was called "aura" healing back in the 1980's. Then I discovered Therapeutic Touch was being taught right in the nursing program and I became so excited. The reality, however, hit when I started working in the hospital as an RN; there just was no time to work with patients on this level. One day I was preparing a very frightened pre-surgery patient who dreaded the procedure. I ended up with a very unhappy operating room (OR) staff because my counseling work with this patient held up their OR schedule. Hospitals are task-oriented, not people-oriented. After seven years I found that the hospital work environment was not well suited for me.

What I yearned for was a safe way to incorporate spiritual and energetic healing for others.

I really wanted to stay in the nursing field and help people on the physical and spiritual levels combined. My studies led me to medical intuitive counseling via a program offered by famed author and medical intuitive Carolyn Myss. Connecting with others felt so important to me in my life's work. Helping people to get in touch with their own intuitive wisdom—to tap into the one heart—was the path I was on. Learning to help people connect with their own intuition and how to listen to their body was my work. I feel if a person goes deep enough they will find the connection to their own deeper issues. In my work I am present as a witness and energetically I hold this space for people to do their own work by creating a safety net to do that.

On a planetary level I feel there is a balancing needed between the divine feminine and the divine masculine. The divine feminine has been suppressed for so many generations. For me to stand in my practice as a woman, I am helping the divine feminine to resurface. This resurfacing of the divine feminine is needed for all living beings.

As women we need to stand in our truth against oppression. Now when I practice as an alternative healer I am standing in my truth.

Babs Smith RN, Certified Intuitive Counselor
American Board of Scientific Medical Intuition.

※

CHAPTER 6

Education of Healing

~⊙~

"A woman healer is as old as history."
~ Mary Chamberlain - author

Modern Healing?

How does western medicine define healing? And when does the healing occur? These are fascinating and important questions to consider.

The word *heal* is derived from the word *hale* or *hal*, which before 900 A.D. meant whole, and is defined as *to make healthy or sound*. Curiously, the word "healing" is less often used in medical circles, with the word *cure* as its replacement. Cure is defined as (1) to restore a person to spiritual wholeness and (2) recovery or relief from a disease.[92]

Do we heal while in the hospital? Often a hospitalized person suffers from lack of sleep due to pain, as well as the hospital procedures and mundane maintenance tasks throughout the day and night. Hospital stays today are relatively short, thanks partly to the insurance industry and Medicare's redesign of diagnostic codes. Healing likely does not take place in the hospital, but somewhere else–perhaps at home or in a nursing home facility.

The lack of yin within institutional walls is evident. The goal of the modern hospital is to "fix" the problem of the patient and then move her out. Fixing is an applicable goal in cases such as an appendectomy or a fractured leg. However, in cases such as heart attack, cancer, stroke, or diabetic complications, what is needed for healing is nurturance and deeper care. And yet since the 1980's, institutional care has become far less nurturing and far more structured, methodical, and inflexible. Abiding by the hospital rules was, and still is, a fixed paradigm.

When we take a further look inside hospitals, we see that they are a training ground, not unlike a battleground, where contests are waged continuously. For example, in Intensive Care Units (ICUs) there is a constant battle for life with patients on the verge of death. The staff must be constantly alert for and ever vigilant of the perceived enemy—death. Even though death is not really the enemy, the fear of this inevitable event absorbs the entire medical staff. Statistics from 2010 reveal that heart disease, cancer, and stroke,[93] the leading causes of death, result as much from poor lifestyle as poor medical care management. The irony of our current health system is that some deaths come from the treatments themselves known as iatrogenic which is a result of the prescriber's treatments (medicines or pharmaceuticals), surgery, or overwhelming antibiotic-resistant infections unique to hospital environments. Exact figures will probably never be known.

The institutional structure with its administrative regulations too often prevents its practitioners from using a holistic perspective. Rather, staff focuses on the patient as a mass of flesh and bones that is given a diagnostic code and a care plan assigned by this code. And the code is, in turn, set by other institutions, namely insurance companies and government Medicare regulators.

Training the Healer

Can healing take place amidst high tension and fear? When creating an environment conducive to healing, what elements are needed? Answering these questions requires a look at both the training environment in medical schools and the major institution for health care itself, the hospital. In my career as a registered nurse (RN), and later as a naturopathic physician (ND), I have listened to stories and complaints from co-workers, peers, and patients. My patients grumbled about being treated in a cold, fast-paced health care setting, while my RN co-workers groused about institutional work environments. Health workers are still leaving their medical profession, especially nurses, for a variety of reasons: lack of respect, little autonomy in the work environment and high workload. The bottom-line profit mentality in patient care and the overly structured hierarchal medical system staffed with often egocentric minds create an unfortunate climate for the patient. Many physicians themselves are unhappy with their insane workloads, where they are often expected to work up to 24-hour shifts, be on call at odd hours, and manage a high patient load (the number of patients to be seen per hour). This burdensome workload has been a long tradition in medicine.

Where does this drive to push doctors and nurses into unforgiving work conditions come from? It begins with the way medical professionals are educated. Ever since medical schools began operation, educating physicians in a sea of high competition has been the norm. Today, to be accepted into a medical school, the premed student must have consistently earned top grades, in most cases nearly a 4.0 average. After the student arrives at medical school, the competition only increases. The pressure is on to maintain high grades to obtain a prestigious residency. Unfortunately, the consistent pressure to make perfect medical decisions affects both the student learner and the patient who is the care recipient. And this high-pressure environment is not limited to training physicians. Other medical professionals such as nurses, nursing assistants, physician assistants, and nurse practitioners are also trained in stressful, hierarchal environments. Rigid adherence to medical dogma and scientific principles prevails in medical training facilities. From there, these priorities are transmitted directly to the patient hospital room. There is little or no room for emotions, feelings, or second-guessing. Feelings by the patient generally are ignored, scoffed at, brushed over, or patronized.

Some hospitals and nursing homes have made attempts to create warmer and homier atmospheres, to counter the common sterile medical environments, and to create at least a superficial sense of deeper caring. But these minor changes cannot bury the patient's fear and the never-ending competition that rules these institutions.

To understand that fear, consider how patients are admitted to a hospital setting; they come in to the hospital either via the emergency department, or at the instruction their own "attending" physician. Additionally, the doctor may recommend elective surgery, other medical treatment, or diagnostic testing. These circumstances often create some feelings of urgency for the patient.

The patient may be worried about the outcome of her hospital stay and wonder what is happening in her body. The hospital staff admits her, interacts on her behalf, and is attentive to her concerns–while also efficiently performing their duties. The staff's primary concern is to follow accurately the "orders" outlined by the doctor. As all this activity occurs around her, the bewildered patient lies on a hospital gurney or sits in a wheelchair. The routines are foreign to her, but business as usual for the staff. Evidence of this business-like approach to patient care is how the staff may talk about the patient as if she were not present. This becomes more pronounced with older patients. Hospital personnel may talk over or speak in loud voices to elders admitted to hospitals, as if the patients were hard of hearing, when really they may just be confused, overwhelmed by this flurry of activity in a new environment, or apprehensive.

Even in the simple process of admitting a patient, there is pressure to get the job done, assuring that this procedure is performed without mistakes. It is imperative to prescribe the right medication, administer the correct IV, or perform the proper diagnostic test, and then monitor that patients move onto their next destination, whether that be the X-ray department, the operating room, the Intensive Care Unit, or the hospital room.

Pressure and urgency is a constant undercurrent in the hospital environment. The staff, usually orderlies, aides, and nurses, know their job well and they work briskly and efficiently to get the job finished. After all, there may be ten more people waiting to be cared for next.

As the newly admitted patient lies in a hospital bed, a new parade of people come into the room to look, examine, palpate, and ask questions over and over, because the admitting staff, the nursing staff, and the physician staff can't seem to get coordinated. The pressure is on to gain insight into the patient's ailment, so as to get it right for the chief physicians, whose inquiries will surely follow. By now, not only the staff, but also the ailing individual is slightly–or more than slightly–anxious.

The word "patient" is a curious term. It is derived from the Latin word "patior," which means to suffer, yet this is the label given to any individual who seeks medical help. "Patient" is defined as "one who is suffering from any disease or behavioral disorder and is under treatment for it."[94] Medical personnel immediately label individuals seeking medical assistance by their disease or diagnosis. Although there has been a movement to name a person seeking medical help as a "client" instead of a "patient," the term "patient" is still in wide use today. Its use may feel demeaning, disconnecting, and disempowering. However, the use of the word "client" has earned mixed reviews. There's no denying, though, that the traditional semantics contributes to the lack of respect for people wearing hospital gowns. After all, in the hospital care of today it is about business; profit is the bottom line.

A Conundrum: Where is the Healing?

Competition between doctors and doctors, doctors and nurses, nurses and nurses, and nurses and supervisors–still prevails in major university and municipal hospital settings on a daily basis, as well as in clinical practices. As you can imagine, this is not conducive to serenity and healing. Originally a hospital was meant to be a place of rest and peace; now they are places of quick treatments with the patient moved onto a rehabilitation or nursing care unit as soon as possible. Hospital culture and purpose has changed over the last 20 years.

Many indigenous cultures have families willing to care for their sick at home and only use hospitals as a last resort for an unmanageable painful death. Love and nurturance at home are what most people, particularly those who are dying, desire. The sick and dying are comforted by their home environment; when they know death is imminent, they often want to die at home, surrounded by loved ones.[95]

Additionally, a study of parents of children who die of cancer reported their family's better post-death adaptation when the death occurred at home rather than in a hospital.[96] Offering care in one's home is a forgotten art, yet before the growth of large medical institutions, home care was commonplace. Home is where the yin resides. Home is our loving environment where true healing can happen. Yin medicine is needed to restore healing to the practice of health care. I believe women know this already and that it should be spoken, clarified, and acknowledged.

The hospice movement that began in the United States in the early 1980s coincided with Dr. Elisabeth Kubler-Ross's profound and thoughtful works on death and dying, which raised the consciousness of both medical professionals and their patients. This was a yin turning point in medicine. Dr. Kubler-Ross asked, "What happens in a changing field of medicine, where we have to ask ourselves whether medicine is to remain a humanitarian and respected profession or a new but depersonalized science in the service of prolonging life rather than diminishing human suffering?" And indeed, have we remained humanized in our health care delivery? From the comments and complaints about it commonly expressed today, I think not.

Having personally witnessed hospital changes from the 1960s to the 1990s, working in ten different hospitals in my career as an RN, I watched the quality of patient care suffer greatly due to staffing decisions based solely on a business model. I found it difficult to remain in a work environment that did not permit professionals like me to render the care that patients deserve. Too often medical staffing decisions were based on the hospital's budget and insurance codes. For sanity and ethical purposes, I left the hospital world over twenty years ago.

Today, nurses work harder and longer hours to meet staffing as well as business requirements. Fewer RNs give direct patient care in the current system; instead the system relies on nursing assistants and specialized technicians to give comfort and nourishment, to monitor and meet the personal needs of patients. Contemporary doctors and nurses now are *technicians* of the human body and the ancillary staff takes care of the patient's personal needs.

My dear friend Judy, also an RN, was scheduled for knee replacement about ten years ago. Intimately familiar with low staffing patterns of hospitals, she diligently set up a family schedule for her post-operative stay in the hospital, knowing that the staff would provide minimal care. Her family rendered the care she needed.

Professional burnout is high among medical profes-sionals. Doctors are stressed to meet the high demand of office and hospital practice. The emergence of the medical specialty called a hospitalist[97] is a response to the overbur-dened schedule of medical doctors. When a hospital utilizes the services of a hospitalist, people admitted into the hospital are no longer cared for by their own familiar doctors, but by a new medical professional whom the patients do not know. The hospitalist may have more focus and updated skills for caring for institutionalized individuals, but how do the patients feel about this new provider whom they have never met? Another stressor for the ailing patient is added to the pile. The hospitalist is a concept that works on paper, but not for the end user—the patient.

The training of medical professionals still includes long hours of work and sleepless nights. Some recent changes reduce the requirement for a resident doctor to stay on duty for 36 hours straight. Sadly, however, this practice is still found in some situations today. The rationale? "It has always been done this way." This is absurd, and should no longer be acceptable. This practice began in earlier times because of a shortage of personnel and many wartime demands. It may have been a necessity to tend to critically ill or injured patients, but how is the safety and protection of the patient built into this system? When ongoing shifts of 24 to 36 hours are the expected norm, the physicians can easily make errors in decision and judgment.

Studies continue to appear about the hazards of the 24- to 36-hour work shifts expected of physicians. An article in the November 2009 issue of the *European Heart Journal* reported that a study of doctors working such extended hours showed irregular heart markers and rhythm.[98] This study indicates the potential dangers of this irrational tradition. The logic of this ongoing practice escapes me.

Medical errors are not well monitored nor documented, so the exact numbers are not known. Recently, Gary Null wrote on the subject of iatrogenic (practitioner-caused) statistics related to deaths within the medical system.[99] Additionally, a book called *Medical Ethics and Conflict of Interest in Scientific Medicine*, published by Jonathan Quick, director of Essential Drugs and Medicines Policy for the World Health Organization (WHO), sheds light on this subject.[100] Community watchdogs report that American medicine can be unsafe and that research around prescribed drugs is flawed.

The following tale is a marvelous example of a woman retaining her intuitive sense and holding onto her power amidst tough medical decisions.

21ˢᵗ Century Tale

Kristin

Kristin Thompson was 37 years old, pregnant for the first time, and thrilled! She and her husband, Chris, had planned for this baby and were preparing to welcome this profound life change. Kristin's first 12 weeks of pregnancy were extremely tough, as she was one of the rare women who experience daylong, unrelenting nausea. So she was excited when the nausea finally subsided at the end of her first three months. She looked forward to her first appointment with the OB/GYN doctor. Her husband accompanied her.

"Hmmm, I need to go get the doctor," said the technician during what should have been a routine ultrasound. Shortly, the technician returned with the doctor, who confirmed the technician's finding: Kristin's young fetus was developing abnormally. The unusual development included a large fluid bubble on the back of his neck (called nuchal translucency). The fluid sac was much, much, larger than usual, the doctor said. The sac was so far out of the range of normal, in fact, that the doctor recommended Kristin have an abortion and "start over."

Kristin and her husband sat, mouths agape, in total shock. The words of the physician echoed in their heads. An abortion? She was 37 years old and had just survived weeks of horrible illness. If she got an abortion, would she be ready and willing to go through twelve weeks of agony again? What if it was too late for second chances? What if she was unable to get pregnant again?

Kristin asked about other options. Her physician advised her to get a CVS, a biopsy to analyze the cells of the placenta, which would tell the couple if there was a chromosomal abnormality. Kristin and Chris immediately opted for the CVS test.

During the visit, a nurse showed them a chart with a variety of percentages: 20% chance of miscarrying, 30% chance of chromosomal disorder, 40% chance of rare genetic disease. The list seemed to go on and on. The nurse told them, "Your child has a 20% chance of being born healthy, normal, or even alive. You should get an abortion."

Devastated once again, Kristin left the room to undergo the biopsy. This was not the pregnancy she had imagined. However, all the pain and devastation was worth it when, a week later, the CVS test came back showing no signs of chromosomal abnormality. It also showed that Kristin and Chris were having a boy!

While this felt like a victory, it was still possible that their baby boy might have any number of other diseases and defects, and because of this the doctors were advising her to terminate the pregnancy. But Kristin had wanted this pregnancy so badly, had suffered weeks of extreme nausea during it, and the thought of starting over horrified her. Besides, her biological clock was ticking. Kristin and Chris thought it might well be this moment or not at all.

As a smart, educated businesswoman, Kristin decided not to take this diagnosis at face value. She went home, hit the computer, and began her own research on the findings noted on the diagnostic screen. Kristin found stories of other mothers who had received the same initial diagnosis, but still given birth to healthy babies. She found *data showing that if ultrasounds showed an otherwise healthy baby and the CVS showed no chromosomal abnormality, all indications were that the baby would be born perfectly fine. This gave Kristin all the hope she needed. She got a referral to a new physician and showed him data that this "indicator" was not necessarily a sentence of death or disability for her baby. The doctor's irritation was palpable, but he agreed to care for her with monthly ultrasounds.*

Admittedly, Kristin and Chris were still terrified. Were they making the right choice? Deep inside, they loved this child and ultimately realized they needed to make decisions about him using the facts they knew for sure and the intuition that had guided them this far.

Kristin delivered a normal, 6 pound 12 ounce baby boy on May 23, 2008. Her son arrived a bit early, at 36 weeks, yet he had a healthy weight and showed no signs of any abnormalities.

Gavin is now a healthy, happy, adorable little boy. His parents feel so blessed that they challenged their doctor's conventional wisdom, advocated on behalf of their unborn child, and followed their intuition to make the right choice for their family.

❧

As this tale illustrates, women know their bodies better than technology does. Kristin was willing to believe her body, trust her intelligence and intuition, and stay in tune with her truth. Women do have innate intuitive abilities; we only have to take the time to tune into them and listen.

CHAPTER 7

Honoring the Feminine Difference

~౨⌒

Women are always being tested... but ultimately each of us
has to define who we are individually and then do the
very best job we can to grow into that.
~Hilary Rodham Clinton

Biological Differences

Recent research has more clearly differentiated women's uniqueness, both physically and emotionally. Historically, women such as Trotula of Salerno and Hildegard of Bingen recorded their findings about female anatomy, but they received little acknowledgment of their work. Recently, however, women have been moving into the medical arena in greater numbers; with this influx comes their questioning spirit. Consequently, researchers have studied female differences; through these efforts medical understanding of the female body is evolving. Throughout history, physicians diagnosed and treated women like they were male bodies and brains. This is obviously not the case.

Dr. Healey was not alone in her focus on and differentiation of women's health from men's health, but because she held a powerful position, she controlled the funding to back her research. However, the sad truth about women's position these last two thousand years is her domination by power and economics. Had a balance of power existed all these years, medical history would certainly read differently. We'd no doubt be familiar with the names Agnodice of Greece, Alice Hamilton, MD, and Mary Putnam Jacobi MD, all of whom changed how medicine was viewed. As women medical practitioners increased in number, concern for the care of underserved populations like the working poor men, women and children became the focus of women in medicine. Many of these practitioners responded to women's cry for a female provider. Women often prefer a female attendant for childbirth and post-childbearing situations; it is easy to understand why, as these experiences are unique to the female body.

Early physicians such as Elizabeth Blackwell, MD; Mary Putnam Jacobi, MD; and Maria Zakrzewska, MD dedicated themselves to providing care to underserved women and their children who were often ignored by male practitioners. Each of these women physicians opened hospitals and clinics to care for these populations in the northeast corridor of the United States. The most famous of these are The New York Infirmary (for Women and Children) founded by Blackwell.[101] Dr. Blackwell's colleague and friend, Dr. Marie Zakrzewska opened and ran a similar hospital in Boston that specialized in gynecology, obstetrics, and pediatrics. History notes that the care women received in these institutes was superior due to the hygienic practices in place. Men at this time were still denying that clean hands or asepsis had any relationship to women's post birth infections.[102]

In the late 19th and early 20th century, women who trained in the female medical colleges traveled West to open clinics in rural America. Some practiced right out of their home kitchens, treating their communities with the best means they had. I honor Dr. Lillie Rosa Minoka Hill (1876-1952), who was inspired by her mother's Mohawk lineage and her father's Quaker beliefs to help others. Dr. Minoka Hill became the Wisconsin Oneida Indian community's first doctor and a favorite among the native people, receiving accolades both from the Oneidas and the Wisconsin Medical Association for her tireless community work.[103]

Women's Experience of Disease

One example of how the medical experiences of women are often misunderstood is a syndrome called Pre-Menstrual Syndrome, most commonly referred to as PMS. This is a collection of symptoms a woman may have 7 to 10 days before the onset of her menstrual cycle. These symptoms may include mood swings, food cravings, headaches, and bloating.

For most of my early medical career, male doctors considered this syndrome a fictitious or psychosomatic complaint. A woman who sought treatment for PMS was placated or ignored. Worse, some doctors treated women as though they had a psychiatric disorder: the standard diagnosis that has evolved for extreme cases is PMDD, or premenstrual dysphoric disorder, classified as a psychiatric condition. Yet in the last 20 years, research has shown that the physiology, specifically hormonal imbalance, is the cause of this syndrome. This research confirms many of the symptoms women experience.

Women also experience a greater incidence of autoimmune disorders such as Rheumatoid Arthritis, Lupus,

Thyroiditis (an inflammatory reaction of the thyroid), and Multiple Sclerosis. Women more often experience these common diseases, yet male doctors predominantly treat them. Another phenomenon that women experience is a syndrome called hypoglycemia, or low blood sugar. Too often, this syndrome received a diagnosis of "It's all in your head, dear." Personally I observed this numerous times in my nursing career.

Now, in my practice as a naturopathic physician, I have learned that these syndromes and others are better under-stood within the context of stress responses and adrenal dysregulation. (The adrenal glands produce hormones in response to environmental and emotional stimuli.) Even today, many of my MD contemporaries do not embrace or understand the physiologic responses and imbalances women often experience. Women simply have different physiologies, and therefore respond in different ways to certain stimuli. In many cases when endocrine hormones are out of balance, restoring the correct hormone balance is all that is needed– not psychotropic drug therapy, the conventional treatment.

The Female Brain

Since 1960, the study of brain physiology has advanced significantly to include the influence of bio-chemicals on brain function. The work of two female researchers, Dr. Cynthia Darlington and Dr. Louann Brizendine, has advanced the knowledge of steroid sex hormones and their influence on the female brain.. Indeed, Dr. Brizendine's work has clar-ified the studies of the female brain, casting light on male and female differences. For instance, while males have some of the same steroid sex hormones (such as estrogen, proges-terone and testosterone), as females do, the proportion and influence of these hormones is significantly different. Furthermore, the hormonal differences start as early as eight weeks into gestation, when female and male physical differentiation begins. Due to this finding, science is now able to monitor the developmental differences in the female brain.

Economics of Health

A review of past societal and medical structures, which cause imbalances in and around health-care delivery, a clearer understanding emerges of the obstacles women have faced, both as recipients and as caregivers. Women have always been caregivers, but history tells us that the economics of health has influenced women's role in healing. Today is little different than the 1500s, when a woman's presence in the health care arena threatened a man's economic value and his livelihood.

To push medicine to exacting limits of understanding, and to create an elitist profession, men have overlooked some important values. The yang values of driving health care by intellect, economics, and rigid science, are spiraling out of control. Medicine should not be doctor-centric, as it has been in the past. Fortunately, a shift has already begun. This shift focuses on placing the patient in the center of a circle and the patient's extended community, including medical professionals, as support within the circle–creating the concept of "patient-centered care."

Putting the patient at the center has always been the intention, I am sure; however, other factors have clouded the original goal. These factors include competition in research, recognition, and achievement; heroic surgical feats to save a life; and medical management based on business practices. In the confusion created by these factors, more has been lost. Medicine has lost its true focus, which is to help patients return to their lives fully recovered–while doing the least amount of harm.

Hippocrates, long honored for his philosophy, would not recognize his teachings today in western medicine. His instructions include, "First, do no harm", and "Let medicine be your food; let food be your medicine." Conventional medicine has not embraced the second of these, and often forgets the first. Hippocrates also wrote about using plants for healing; pharmaceutical medicines hardly resemble most plants today. The growth of the drug industry has expanded mostly due to great marketing. I, first hand, know the value of appropriate life-saving pharmacology. However prescribing multiple drugs for one person is dangerous at best. This concern has been raised in medical circles, but multiple drug prescribing continues. Often the second or third drug added is to mitigate side effects of an earlier prescription. When a medical practitioner is educated in one or two treatment modalities (drugs and surgery), their options are limited.

Medicine needs to incorporate the ease and flow of yin, to restore balance through an extended healing process, to honor patient-centered health care. This type of health care requires communication among all parties involved in the person's care and carefully, selectively prescribing supportive treatments. Women have a deep gift of community and communication with one another, as research into women's brains and social lives has repeatedly shown; women are ideally suited for this yin type of health care.

New ideas are coming to light, however to help patients and doctors communicate better. It is a great relief to know about the "The Society of Participatory Medicine." This non-profit organization states: "Participatory Medicine is a movement in which networked patients shift from being mere passengers to responsible drivers of their health, and in which providers encourage and value them as full partners."[104]

As the lines of communication open wider and deeper, healing can really happen.

Women's Voice

The value of women speaking out medical matters has historically been challenged. In a few cultures she has been revered; in western culture she is not revered in the way she deserves. Unfortunately, what remains is the fact that the thinking, reasoning, and intuitive voice of women has been sidelined . In the operating room, in the patient room and in medical schools, women's contributions have been largely ignored or belittled. My career observations confirm this fact.

Few texts on the history of medicine are written from the feminine perspective or even in her voice . Yet women experience life, sickness, and death very differently than men do. This is not to say that men's perspective is not good, but rather that women's perspective is closer to the emotional and intuitive level. That perspective is just as good–but different. I believe it is time to recognize, welcome, and incorporate the feminine perspective. I believe it is this perspective that gives us the introspection, balance, kindness, joy, contentment, and love we all want to experience in reaching health and wholeness. Again bring yin to interconnect with the yang.

Since about the year 2000, women's voices in medical research have become more prominent. As more women enter the medical field and move into research, the bias is changing. Cynthia Darlington, PhD, writes in *The Female Brain,*

"In terms of scientific development, the investigation of the female brain is only at the very beginning of the process. There are a lot more disparate pieces of information to be analyzed."[105]

As a researcher, Darlington clearly points out the influence of hormones, not only on the brain (the organ they most affect), but also in the way they affect women when multiple drug therapies are prescribed. Estrogen and progesterone have specific receptors throughout the body; the way these hormones chemically respond to pharmaceuticals is only now being discovered. Fluctuations in the levels of these and other hormones can further influence responses to prescribed medicines.[106]

Female Response to Stress

Women respond differently than men to stressful events. Recent studies of oxytocin[107] document this difference. Dr. Brizendine, writes that women do not always use the well-known fight-or-flight response that males often favor. Instead, a female may prefer bonding and social contact, or she may prefer avoiding conflict in the first place[108]. In studies of female animals, once they have bonded with their young, females prefer to stay and protect them, even when in danger. Other females often come to offer assistance or sound alerts in a stressful or threatening situation. This pattern of behavior, called "trend and befriend," often occurs in female groups.[109] Teenage girls often display a similar behavior, bonding with one another, sometimes intensely, once they begin to produce ovarian estrogen. Stimulated by estrogen, oxytocin is the primary female brain hormone; it is released when a woman falls in love. The counterpart male hormone is vasopressin. Each has different effects, reports Dr. Brizendine, but both hormones affect the brain chemical dopamine, the "feel good" brain chemical.[110]

Laura Cousino Klein, PhD, and Shelley Taylor, PhD, reported further confirmation of female bonding in a 2000 UCLA study. They believe that omitting women from stress research has been a huge mistake. Women tend to bond with one another, sharing their thoughts and emotions. This social skill often begins in the teenage years and serves woman throughout her life.[111]

Is Death a Failure?

Elizabeth Kubler-Ross, MD, and Cicely Saunders, MD, are the two women who taught us how to honor death–a true yin quality. Dr. Kubler-Ross was trained as a psychiatrist and authored the ground breaking best seller, *On Death and Dying,*, in 1969. She is known internationally for her work, which focused on spending time listening to dying patients talk of their lives, fears, and anxieties. Dr. Kubler-Ross came to the US in 1958 and was appalled at the treatment this patient population received; she felt that the medical professional shunned and abused them, that no one was honest with them. She is quoted saying, "My goal was to break through the layer of professional denial that prohibited patients from airing their inner-most concerns...[112] and went on to write over twenty books on the subject; they have been translated into more than twenty-five languages. She is also the recipient of more than twenty honorary doctorates.

I had the great honor to meet this woman in 1982. I felt her mesmerize an audience for hours with her passionate tales filled with a sense of hope. What she brought to dying individuals was the affirmation that they were valuable, that others were listening to them, and that they would not be forgotten. Her words were comforting for me as a hospice nurse working in a specialty newly arrived in the U.S.

In our current model of saving lives at all cost, medicine has lost sight of accepting the end of life. For those who believe in life after death, death is but a new experience on the journey. Unfortunately, though, the yang approach to medicine rebuffs the idea of allowing death to proceed as a natural occurrence. But, no matter what, death will take place. Medicine can prolong the dying process via such machines as heart pumps, electrical stimulators, and ventilators, but the greater wisdom may be simply to allow it to take place, accepting what is inevitable.

In the military medical paradigm, death is not seen as an option for a young, injured soldier. And, indeed, giving encouragement and support at critical moments offers the hope of survival to the injured. This makes perfect sense in a frantic, life-saving moment. But does it make sense when the scenario concerns chronic illnesses or devastating metastatic cancers? Not as much. In these instances, preparing for death is a dignified approach to life.

Cicely Saunders, MD, worked with dying patients in the UK who were left alone to die in institutions. She felt a great need to comfort and care for these individuals. As she came to understand her dying patients, she developed protocols for pain relief with opiates, which greatly relieved a patient's anxiety and fears.[113] "Often their suffering is intensified by isolation and loneliness," Saunders reported. Because of these experiences, Saunders raised significant funds to open St. Christopher's, Britain's first hospice. This facility was the model for the hospice movement that eventually found its way to America in the early 1980s. When Saunders was awarded a one million dollar grant to continue her work, she said, "This award recognizes how science and humanity need to go together and that is what hospices are all about."[114]

As an emergency room (ER) nurse, I witnessed many deaths during my career. People either came into the hospital already dead (DOA), or arrived in the ER where resuscitation efforts were unsuccessful. These were hard times, not only for the patient's family, but also for the ER staff. The attending ER doctor had the job of pronouncing the death and then reporting it to loved ones. The sudden loss always brought outbursts of emotions that were difficult for others to witness. As the dutiful nurse, it was my job to procure and administer a sedative to the grieving family. And yet, it was always a puzzle to me why we suppressed grief in this manner. Who was the sedative really for–the grief-stricken family or those who felt discomfort watching her? In my mind, grief and loss are but a part of the cycle of life.

When a life is lost during a heroic medical moment, it may feel like failure. This attitude, however, is clearly a yang attitude. While admirable in concept, it needs to be rethought. Death is not a failure at all, especially when all human effort has been made to prevent it. At such moments it is important to remember yin and yang as a healing concept. The cycle of life includes the beginning and ending of life as we know it. It is a natural occurrence, a natural balance, a natural flow. It happens in nature and it happens in human life.

The word *compassion* must be brought into the equation: compassion for the rescuers as well as compassion for the rescued. Police, fire fighters, EMT's (Emergency Medical Technician), 911 dispatchers, and medical staff who are attracted to the role of rescuer, whether on a battlefield, in a burning building, or at a horrific traffic accident, need self-compassion along with unwavering support. They perform their roles and duties as best as they can in the moment. I have witnessed some of the harshest and cruelest criticisms in the health-care world meted out to hard, overworked medical staff. A gaping hole exists in the current medical health-care system: inadequate support, compassion, and understanding for the day-to-day demands and stresses of performing life-saving skills unfailingly. Danielle Ofri, MD, shares poignant patient-doctor stories from her ten years at Bellevue Hospital in New York City. She conveys her feelings during the many difficult, challenging medical situations, and concludes by saying she cried for the loss of many of her cases but also, "I cried for the death of my belief that intellect conquers all."[115]

Self-compassion lessens the tension when healers are helping the sick and dying, and allows for more presence with those in their care. An institutional setting should offer the same level of compassion for the healers as for the sick and dying. Individuals dedicated to performing care-giving roles need to examine the set of rules under which they function. Being kind and compassionate first to oneself needs to be the highest priority. What drives practitioners in their work is a good place to start the self-examination. Unfortunately, this introspective approach is not taught in medical school, nor is it supported by institutional administrations.

21st Century Tale

Nancy

Nancy was 58 years old, a vibrant woman who loved to dance, sing, and hike. She had studied in California with Herman Aihara, one of the great macrobiotic teachers, and followed a macrobiotic lifestyle. During the course of her illness she followed a traditional Ayurvedic healing regimen.

I knew Nancy for several years before we each separately moved to the Pacific Northwest. Nancy and I shared many common interests, which we talked about for hours. We also were part of a women's spiritual circle that met weekly. During those years, our circle of women shared both tears and laughter, resulting in a deep closeness. We became sisters with a spiritual bond that none of us had experienced before. It was magical. It was healing.

And then Nancy was diagnosed with breast cancer in her right breast. She spent several weeks in contemplation and soul-searching to determine her treatment regimen. Finally, she decided–she would have surgery. Because the cancer had spread to five (of nine) lymph nodes, the nodes and her right breast were removed.

Following the surgery, Nancy decided on her own course of treatment. There would be no chemotherapy, no radiation. She chose her own plan for her life. Nancy was now on an unknown journey and we supported her decision. We were a part of her.

About two years after her initial diagnosis, Nancy's energy sagged; the cancer was advancing. When she could no longer manage well on her own, she had a hospital bed and commode delivered to her home. Meanwhile, Nancy prepared for her passage. She hired a spiritual facilitator and at her invitation we all participated in a spiritual prayer circle. We read from the Tibetan Book of the Living and the Dying.[116] We chanted and shared together in her living room. This was Nancy's prayer.

In November our group, along with family and friends, celebrated Nancy's 60th birthday. During this big celebration of her life, she gave away some of her precious belongings to those who felt moved to cherish something of hers. I chose a round Korean drum that I still play today, reminding me of our friendship.

In her final days, I sat with her, as she wished, staying with her so she would not be alone. Lovingly, I held her hand to my heart. It was an honor to be a witness to this intentional journey. On the day she died, our sister circle gathered around. Together we bathed her, sang, and dressed her in her best ceremonial clothing. After her death, we followed the Tibetan Buddhist tradition of not removing her body for 24 hours. My friend and spiritual sister Babs and I held vigil for those hours until her body was removed. As Nancy was carried out her front door, we drummed her spirit to fly away safely to her next life.

Death is not the enemy. Death has wings.

CHAPTER 8

Bringing Balance Back

~◎~

"For to be a woman is to have interests and duties, raying out in all directions from the central mother core, like spokes from the hub of a wheel. The pattern of our lives is essentially circular. We must be open to all points of the compass: husband, children, friend, home, community; stretched out, exposed, sensitive like a spider's web to each breeze that blows, to each call that comes."
~ Anne Morrow Lindbergh

Feminine Healing Takes its Place

In most cases, healing does not happen spontaneously, or even quickly. Surgeries may stop hemorrhaging, repair traumatic injuries, or remove diseased tissue, but true, deep healing takes much longer. This is because healing is different from curing. Healing involves the integration of the physical, the emotional, and the spiritual energies of the body. Curing is defined as a successful remedial treatment; it is a "fix" for a disease or getting rid of something detrimental.[117]

Healing contains yin quality; cure contains yang quality.

The idea of separating the mind from the body when treating any medical condition never made sense to me. Whether it is a traumatic injury or a long term chronic disease, the mind and emotions play a significant role in outcome/recovery. When science took a dominant place in medical training, the separation of the physical from the intellectual and emotional created a chasm. When I speak to women colleagues about this separation we usually agree that you cannot treat the body without also involving the mind and emotions. My male colleagues often realize this, too, but in the modern medical system the separation still exists.

Eliza Lo Chin, MD, collected essays and poems by contemporary female physicians, capturing how women have moved into medicine and are attempting to right the balance of a heavily male-oriented system.[118] Their efforts have not been easy. They report having to endure insults, sexism, and a blatant lack of support from their male colleagues. Story after story in Lo Chin's book reveals this seamy side of medicine. Yet, women have persisted. And with the help of Title IX[119], the law passed in 1972 that lifted sexist barriers, more women have become physicians. Today, female medical students are on par in numbers with males.[120]

In an article published in the *New York Times*, Pauline Chen, MD, explores whether men or women make better physicians. She writes that even male patients prefer female doctors, who pay more attention and take more time to listen. A recent article on patient-doctor relations in the *Journal of American Medical Association (JAMA)* reports a similar conclusion: "Female primary care physicians engage in more communication that can be considered patient centered and have longer visits than their male colleagues."[121]

The evidence is clear: women have an important place

in the medical arena. Medicine is being infused with feminine energy, a fact shown by the increasing number of female medical school students. However, statistics show that women still do not hold positions of power in the medical hierarchy. Men still hold most prestigious academic positions, and hospitals run as businesses using a corporate model. Both men and women have administrative hospital positions, however, the business model is yang oriented.

Uniquely Feminine

Every woman needs to appreciate her own unique physiology. It is different and normal–female normal. The medical world is finally coming to appreciate the uniqueness of a woman's body. As research continues to study the female body and uncover both its nuances and its differences, women are coming to know their worth and power. The yang energy telling us what to do with our bodies has disempowered us for too long.

Women are cyclic and rhythmic; we wax and wane just like the moon. We exist in the flow of life. As we let our body fluids flow like rivers, we can change and reshape our lives into what we truly want to be. Even in menopause, our rhythms continue to the end of life. Biorhythms of our body hormones, combined with neurotransmitters and enzymatic activities, have a purpose creating our feminine uniqueness. These complex systems create who we are; we can befriend these rhythms and go with them. Instead of medicating or suppressing these hormones, we need to understand them, honor them, and know their power.

In many western cultures women have learned to turn off their senses and sensibilities. We need to bring these to the forefront once again and put them in the center of our being. We've stopped trusting our senses; we have favored scientific data exclusive of softer qualities, limiting input from the yin side. In the medical setting, both scientific research and intuitive senses need to have a balanced place in decisions affecting a patient's life.

The current dominance of the scientific over the intuitive is no more egalitarian than supplying food only to blue-eyed people would be! There is no democracy in medicine. How we choose to walk through our illnesses, our aging process, and our own death is our privilege and it needs to be our choice in health care. In life's journey, no one gets out alive. In truth physicians do not have all the answers. And that needs to be all right. I think we need to relieve physicians of the burden of always getting it right. Medicine need not be seen as a contest or a trial. In some medical circles, conquering a disease is equated to winning a war, except in war or no war, human lives have more dimension. As complex beings on a journey of unknown length, some need more help than others. Perhaps the practitioner could ask, "What is it you would like?"

An Intuitive Healer

I greatly admire a woman from New South Whales in the Australian outback. Elizabeth Kenny was an informally trained nurse and cared for people in outlying communities where medical care was scarce. This is a story not only of courage, but also of conviction, and of a healing method that she knew worked.

An epidemic of polio broke out in her area. Known than as a "bush" nurse, she tended the young children and developed a method of treatment that resulted in remarkable disease recovery. Poliomyelitis is a disease caused by a virus that attacks the spinal cord, resulting in various degrees of paralysis. Her healing method involved nutrition, a series of hot packs to the affected limbs, and gentle exercise and massage. Eventually her work came to the attention of the Australian government and Elizabeth Kenny was subsequently invited to U.S. to teach her methods. By this time she was honored with the title "Sister," a British title denoting chief nurse. At first she was not well received by the U.S. medical profession; her treatment methods were controversial. Most MD's used boards and braces to treat polio patients. But she persisted with her method and toured the U.S. helping children and adults. Some reports say she had up to an 80% recovery rate. And she did not charge for her services.

She received numerous awards for her independent, courageous work. At the University of Minnesota orthopedic doctors studied her methods; the results of her simple treatments had significantly better outcomes than the then-standard methods of treatment. Polio was a devastating illness; this woman healer understood that simple methods worked. She had no formal medical training, yet was recognized for her intuitive natural methods. Her work became known as the Sister Kenny Method. Accolades bestowed on her in the 1940's made her one of the most popular women in American, on par with Eleanor Roosevelt.

Achieving Yin and Yang Balance

How do we bring healing back into balance with today's yang medical perspective? Massage and heat packs were yin methods in Sister Kenny's work, compared with the steel braces and wooden boards of conventional methods.

The causes of medical yang imbalance are certainly multifaceted, but reviewing the history of western medicine shows how contemporary medicine is built on an uncompromising, structured model. Qualities of yang dominate when making hurried surgical decisions, prescribing only drug-based therapies, blindly following doctor's orders, offering a seven-and-a-half minute office visit, and telling patients that only a medical professional knows what is right for them.

For the medical men of an earlier era, the military world offered a familiar and organized system that worked efficiently to get things done. Its system of delivering medical care worked: a quick response saved lives in many dire situations. Even Florence Nightingale used this system to implement sanitary procedures and standard protocols for the sick and dying in military hospitals. The model is useful, but it is not the only way to deliver health care; so much more is possible.

Clearly now in the twenty-first century, this old system needs revamping and upgrading to restore a balance of yin and yang. For this to happen, certain principles must change.

Medical training needs to include the importance of empathy, listening skills, and including patients and their family in determining a care plan. The word "ego" doesn't not belong beside the title of doctor. A physician needs to be just another member of the health care team. The focus needs to be on healing and on respect for the patients. This includes respect for the patients' ideas and contributions to their own healing process. Often, a person seeking help for a health problem has some good clues on causes and possible cures; these ideas need to be heard and considered.

A recent hospital study showed people with many frequent visitors recovered faster and went home sooner than those who had few or no visitors and little family support.[122] A hospitalized patient can feel isolated and out of touch with the outside world. Hospital visiting rules have relaxed considerably in the last few years, but hospitals still hold control. This is particularly true in intensive care units, coronary care units, and emergency departments, where control of visitors is still tightly regulated. People on the edge of life need their loved ones nearby, to hold them, to reassure or sing to them, either urging them back to wellness or releasing them to death. In what may be their last hours on earth, patients have a right to be with their loved ones.

The stoic professional model taught to young physicians needs to incorporate more compassion and humanity. Too often medical personnel feel they cannot express their feelings or show emotions, as it would just not be "professional." The result is what appears to be an aloof practitioner who hesitates to become involved, just the opposite of what is needed. As both a registered nurse and a physician, I have been compassionate without being overwhelmed by the patient's medical dilemma. It is good to show our caring side to patients; while not always easy, we can separate our feelings from the patient's. Compassion and nurturing are yin qualities that have a place in the medical setting.

Principles of Healing

There are basic guiding principles that describe how the body heals itself. Hippocrates spoke of them in his philosophy. The first essential tenet of healing is *Vis Medicatrix Naturae,* which translates as "the healing power of nature." It addresses the self-healing power that is part of the body's innate intelligence. L. Frank Schnell, MD, further defines it when he says, "Once injury or disease has occurred, the body brings into play its reparative or healing forces under the direction of the autonomic nervous system. "[123]

The principle of *Primum non nocere*, or "first, do no harm", also comes from Hippocrates and should be applied to those who are sick or suffering. The medical treatments we deliver need to be supportive, gentle, and healing. However, the treatments I observed during my many years of nursing were often in direct contradiction to this tenet. Some of the popular yin therapies today include such disciplines as homeopathic medicine, energy medicine, and hands-on body work. Women today still prefer supportive, nurturing care for themselves and their families, especially their children.

"Treat the whole body" – *Tolle Totum*, is another essential belief about how well the body is connected. An injured extremity, for example, calls upon the inflammatory response of the endocrine (hormone) and immune systems, along with the nervous system especially if there is pain involved. How a person responds to the injury, how it affects her lifestyle and how it will prevent her from working or caring for her family all play a part. It is a whole body experience; almost any injury or sickness has an impact on the mind. The powerful mind is a major player in the recovery process. Current medical focus of attending to only the injured part or the "diseased" part is folly. The body is more than a machine in need of replacement parts; too often contemporary medical practice separates the body, mind, and spirit experience.

The well known "placebo effect", documented consistently in medical research since the 1960's, illustrates the power of the mind-body connection. About 30% of research subjects who are given a placebo experience real improvement in their conditions.[124]

Yes, you can replace body parts successfully, but can you heal completely without the power of love, nurturance, and intention? Many men and women return from active military duty physically intact, but often struggle with post traumatic stress disorder (PTSD). They may suffer through years of psychological disability because their minds and spirits have not healed. When disease occurs, it encompasses and affects all of the human being, including mind, body, and spirit. These three aspects cannot be separated; they are, in fact, interwoven, like a web. Put simply, I believe everything is connected to everything.

Medical case studies include numerous stories of people who receive an organ transplant from a deceased donor and begin to experience new cravings. In many cases the deceased organ donor often had these feelings. How is this explained? It is one of the mysteries of yin.

And this leads to another important healing principle, that of *Tolle causum*, or "treat the cause." Because everything is connected in the body, identifying the cause of the disease at its origin makes more sense than identifying how symptoms are manifesting. In moving from an allopathic registered nurse to a naturopathic physician, my medical view has completely changed. Finding the cause of an illness is like playing detective and it is satisfying to discuss possible causes with my patient. This brings the focus back to the patient, placed at the center of her care.

The yin may not be readily quantified; yet it does exist.

Simple Remedies Reborn

Can simple remedies, such as rest, sunshine, relaxation, water, and good nutrition, be too simple to be effective? In truth, bathing and resting are two of the greatest healers of all time. Both have been practiced for thousands of years by millions of people. Both can heal with what is known as the "tincture of time." In today's harried and frenetic culture, these simple modalities are too often overlooked. People claim that their "insurance doesn't cover that," which means it is not sanctioned by the medical industry, and therefore is interpreted as ineffective. But in many cases, performing the simplest self-care treatment can be as good as or better than drug therapy.

Just because a therapy is simple does not mean it does not work. I am a big proponent of trying the simple first–always. Water therapies can be as simple as relaxing in a stress-reducing bath or soaking in the rich mineral waters of hot springs found in many places all over the globe. It can be soaking an injured extremity in alternately warm and cool baths to help repair damaged cells. Extensive research done in many European countries confirms the medicinal value of mineral springs for chronic conditions such as arthritis and back pain. The effectiveness of a homeopathic remedy cannot be overstated here. Personally I have received homeopathic remedies, and have offered homeopathic remedies that are life-changing. The placebo effect is not in play as these remedies work for children and animals with significant effectiveness.

Nutrition is another simple healer that is often overlooked in conventional medical training. The United States has a huge disaster on its hands, simply because its population has a poor understanding of the critical role food plays in everyday health. While the medical profession stood silently by, the food industry hijacked knowledge of good nutrition, by telling the public what to eat. The medical industry seems to believe that what it does not study, research, and sanction has no value. Physicians do not receive nutrition education in their medical training. They learn a bit about vitamins, but that is not nutrition. Because the medical profession partners with the United States government, it has powerfully influenced the public. Allopathic medicine has neglected to teach the public the value of eating simple, whole, and healthy foods. The food we buy, prepare, and feed our families is essential to healthy survival of a nation. Women have known this for centuries, but the mass marketing tactics of the modern food industry, a very yang paradigm, supplanted their knowledge. Americans are dying of preventable heart disease and diabetes, due to this tragic parlay of power.

Just as with water and rest, our foods need to be simple, too. Michael Pollan, a medical journalist, titled his article, *Eat Food, Not Too Much, Mostly Plants*.[125] Consuming fewer processed foods and less sugar, along with more fruits and vegetables, would resolve the major health crisis we are now facing. Mr. Pollan lectures and writes that we need to get back to food basics. And we do.

There is still a need for advanced and complex medical interventions along with good public health policies to prevent epidemics; we are living in a more toxic, polluted environment, and people are sicker than ever before. The healing process starts by restoring the yin ways of healing. First, use simple remedies, balance stress and collaborate with a team of healthy providers, Seek the advice of a healer who knows the body's innate ability; work together to restore and regenerate through cleansing and supportive body care systems.

Teach the Healers

Docere, the Latin word from which *doctor* is derived, means "to teach," or "doctor as teacher." It is defined as one of the three guiding principles of functional and natural medicine.[126] Functional medicine addresses the underlying causes of disease, using a systems-oriented approach and engaging both the patient and practitioner in a therapeutic partnership.[127]

Those of us in the medical profession need to teach others about the simple ways to heal, such as eating healthy and nutritious foods, getting a good night's sleep, relaxing to rebuild and restore our trillions of cells, using water as a healing tool, and soaking in fresh air and sunshine as immune support. These simple treasures, along with plant medicines, homeopathic remedies, and lifestyle changes, have the ability to heal when we know how to use them accurately and thoughtfully.

"Physician, heal thyself," is often bantered about in medicine. My observations over the last forty-plus years tell me that medical workers do a poor job of caring for themselves. Caseloads are large, hours are long, stress levels run high, and poor nutrition is rampant. Typical foods found in doctor's clinics and hospital break rooms are sugary or salty snacks of donuts, candy bars, chips, coffee, and soda pop. During times of high stress, these foods answer the emergency demand for cortisol, a major stress hormone. Over time, however, these same foods contribute to caregivers' succumbing to illnesses similar to their patients.

Healing oneself requires going inside to listen and to give oneself compassion. Women in general freely give to others before giving themselves the care they need. It is an expected role that women fulfill worldwide. Barbara Ehrenreich, a journalist who has written books and articles about women workers, writes about her vision of, "...society in which healing is not a commodity distributed according to the dictates of profit but is integral to the network of community life...in which wisdom about daily life is not hoarded by 'experts' or doled out as a commodity, but is drawn from the experience of all people and freely shared among them."[128] This is a reminder of why many of us come to the healing arts: to share with one another the knowledge, wisdom, and connection that increases our capacity for healing others.

Understanding the true healing aspects of medicine, which include the innate capacities of nature *and* nurture, underscores the appropriateness of a medical system with both yin and yang values. Doctors are people, with the same needs as anyone else: to be whole, accepted, and respected in their work every day. We must help let the façade fall away; remove the perception that doctors, nurses, and other health providers have a better understanding of life. They don't. The imbalance that has been created by too much yang energy can right itself by welcoming in the yin. Honoring both aspects of the whole, owning that yin holds an equal status with yang, will right the balance.

This imbalance is not a new phenomenon. Over one hundred years ago, Sarah Adamson Dolley, MD, wrote, *In all departures of health of body, mind or spirit, I believe there is a loss of balance. Though we may have other terms, harmony equilibrium, etc., the point and principle of getting righted...must be to restore that balance.*

A Deeper Look at Yin: Woman's Innate Nature

What is innate and what is your nature? Innate nature describes those qualities found in every living being, those qualities we are born with. Too many times the naturalness of children is taught out of them. Children's natural curiosity, playfulness, sensitivity to external stimulus, connectedness, sweetness, and kindness change over the young years to become what is considered socially acceptable. In other words we lose our natural way of being with one another and ourselves.

Returning to yin or one's innate nature is the process of going back to some of the innocent qualities lost to cultural norms long ago. These qualities remind us of the authentic self. Gabor Mate, M.D.[129] talks about two essential needs, after food and shelter, that a human infant has: attachment and authenticity. As health providers we perform at our best when we are authentic with our client. Too often our professional persona prevents this authenticity with those we work with. Practicing with yin means returning to our authentic selves.

21st Century Tale

Charlotte

My grown son landed in the hospital when an infection from a cat bite on his finger turned virulent and spread up his arm and through his lymphatic system. He'd done everything right after the initial accident, seeing the doctor for what he thought was a cat scratch and a sprained finger. But as his hand swelled, and later as red streaks appeared up his arm, it became evident that this injury was far more than a sprained and scratched finger.

As a mother, it was terrifying to watch the progress of his infection. The sight of my big, handsome, strong son lying immobilized in a hospital bed was surreal. On the second night, after he'd had a constant stream of IV antibiotics pumped into him, his infection was getting worse, not better. I started to really fret then. I wondered: what would happen if the infection got out of control? Would they amputate his arm? As the days passed and the medical staff told him he would have to stay in the hospital yet another day, the seriousness of his situation hit me. Most of the time hospitals kick patients out as fast as they can. I'd taken my husband home shortly after ear surgery with a bandage wrapped around his head and blood seeping through it. Yet they were insisting, day after day, that my son stay.

He ended up staying in the hospital for five long days, and ultimately needed surgery to scour the infection out of his knuckle. Overall, he got great care, and I'm certain that 21st century medicine and the hospital staff saved his life. Not being the type of family who has ever had much to do with hospitals (the staff couldn't believe this was his first hospital stay), it was fascinating to observe the routines of the institution.

The first thing that became clear was that the nurses do all the real patient care, and they do it well. To a person, they were attentive, caring, and helpful. The doctors, on the other hand, seemed rushed and distant. My son's designated hospitalist changed mid-stay and the second one admitted he was at a loss how to judge my son's situation, since he'd come to the case mid-stream. This same doctor swore every visit that he'd be in early the next morning, yet never showed up until late afternoon.

Similarly, we waited all day for a visit from the surgeon and when she finally showed up, she quickly deemed his hand too swollen to be examined and left, saying she'd be back the next day. That was the last we saw of her until the morning of his actual surgery, several days later.

Communication between doctors and nurses followed similar patterns. My son waited all day in terrible pain for a nurse to get permission from the doctor to increase his meds. The night before his surgery, none of his nurses seemed to know that he was being operated on in the morning, and my son had to warn them not to give him water after midnight. There was little to no communication between the hospitalist and the surgeon, with each seemingly operating in a different sphere. This was worrisome, to say the least. If they didn't even know he was scheduled for surgery, how would the operation itself progress?

Surgery, however, was quick and efficient, once they figured out he was scheduled for it. He was back in his room a couple of hours later, and it occurred to me that aggressive interventions are the type of things that modern-day hospitals do best.

I'm grateful for the care he received and thankful he has retained the use of his arm. And I still can't help but wonder if it all could have been prevented had his original doctor taken just a bit more time and care to ascertain that his injury was a toxic cat bite rather than a simple scratch. It felt as if some of the balance was left out.

Charlotte Rains Dixon

CHAPTER 9

Healing Solutions: A Place to Begin

~ාන

Learn to get in touch with the silence within yourself. There's no need to go to India or somewhere else to find peace. You will find it in your room, your garden, or even in your bathtub.

~Elisabeth Kubler-Ross, MD

Your Intuitive Senses

Intuition is an integral part of every human being on the planet. We are all born with it. There is no one without it. Children are born naturally intuitive. However, in western cultures their innocence, sensitivities, and natural sense of wonder are too often pushed aside, ridiculed, or simply ignored. The ongoing acculturation of children ensures that they follow the norms of their society. Making money, climbing the proverbial ladder, attaining academic accolades, thrill-seeking adventures, and other fast-paced options take precedence in a yang culture. When life is full of yang distractions, there is less time or room for yin.

Being in touch with our own intuitive state of being should come before we embark on a crusade to help others. Intuition is the natural knowing that comes from inside us, and it is the antithesis of science. Like yin, intuition is also the antithesis of yang. For example, one instinctual part that gets shut down in this process is sensing danger. Children are instinctively repelled by certain objects or places. This instinct comes from their inner knowing. It is different than fear, which comes from an irrational belief. This acronym says it best: FEAR = False Evidence Appearing Real. Instinct and intuition are not connected to fear.

Intuition is defined as "direct perception of truth, fact independent of any reasoning process."[130] Contrast this to science, which uses exacting steps and processes to reach rational conclusions, and only accepts what can be undeniably proven.

Intuition and science have been at odds since science emerged hundreds of years ago. The truth is that they are both correct and important for one another. Both have an important side-by-side place in medicine. They are not mutually exclusive. The split of pure scientific proof from the power of the mind and spirit has been a huge detriment to medicine. The human body is clearly one whole entity and operates like yin and yang. One is part of the other.

Helping others in their quest for health and wellness as they recover from an illness or a trauma is a noble profession. However, it is also important that we, as healers, look at our own motives. We must not only appreciate our passion for coming to the aid of others; we must examine it as well. By reflecting on the reason we choose to do our work, we can begin to bring ourselves more into balance. In turn as we follow our intuitive senses, our work becomes authentic;

people who receive care from an intuitive authentic practitioner benefit.

Medical Dichotomy

I witnessed the dichotomy in medicine with the separation of mind (mental illness) from the body (physical illness) first-hand in the 1960s as a young woman in a large metropolitan hospital center in New York City. Yet this split is still functioning in much the same way, fifty years later. If you have a physical disease, medical insurance will cover it. But if you have a mental or emotional disease, insurance benefits are very often limited or not available. Why would this be? Both are classified as illnesses and both deserve full treatment. It is better understood today that our emotional state has an impact on our physical illness, which is demonstrated by the presence of stress-related diagnoses. One common example is depression; once this diagnosis appears in a medical record, the sufferer may not be insurable in the future. Yet depression can be but one of a collection of symptoms associated with thyroid disease or other hormonal imbalances – a physical disturbance.

In the article *Going to the Heart of the Matter; do negative emotions cause heart disease?* the abstract states, "Negative emotions, such as anger, anxiety, and depression, have emerged as potentially important risk factors for coronary heart disease"[131]. Men often die earlier than women; these early deaths may be related to life pressures that have no outlet. Stressful situations also aggravate disturbances of the digestive tract such as peptic ulcers and irritable bowel syndrome (IBS). In my professional career, many of my patients report that disease onset occurred after a major life event such as an accident, divorce, or death of a loved one. We are integrally related. Emotions and illnesses are intertwined. It may be difficult to see clearly where the interconnection lies, but by asking questions and remaining authentic, answers will usually come.

A Yin Approach

In a yin team approach the patient is treated as a whole person and not just as a liver transplant, a hip replacement, or a heart attack. Restoring our current medical system means closing the gap between mental/emotional illness and physical illness. It also includes the patient's input and knowledge as valuable and relevant. A place to begin improving medical care is by starting with the basics of self care, teaching healthy lifestyles, and positively believing that health can be restored to the body.

CHAPTER 10

For Provider and Patient – A New Approach

~⊙~

"There is nothing worse than a sharp image of a fuzzy concept."
~ Ansel Adams

What Can Be Offered?

As a care provider the questions you must answer are two: What do you want in your work career? What are your motives for helping others?

As you answer these questions, be authentic and clear. How satisfied are you with your work? What feeds your soul? Understanding your work motivations can give you insights to help you continue in such a demanding profession. Clarity of purpose will lead to greater satisfaction in your current career, or offer insights about making changes to achieve more contentment.

As a patient in the health care system, particularly if your condition is chronic over many years, the questions to ask are these: What do I need? How well do I understand my life's purpose and where does my illness fit in?

In your answer be authentic and clear.

A balanced doctor-patient relationship needs to be authentic and clear for both parties. Patients must ask for what they need to become well. Women in particular are reluctant to ask for what they *really* need or want. Women are usually comfortable in a giving role, and less often in a receiving one. Sometimes women feel helpless: helpless to make changes, helpless to feel they can be proactive, and helpless to speak out. Martin Seligman, PhD, first developed the learned helplessness theory while working with dogs. Helplessness occurs when animals or humans repeatedly find themselves in a situation that appears hopeless; after several failed attempts, they give up trying to change the situation. Women have learned helplessness through repeated experiences as second-class citizens. Women have more limitations and fewer opportunities than their male counterparts, and often give up trying to change situations. Thus the status quo is maintained: because a woman expects less, she receives less.

By asking a patient what she wants, needs, and expects to receive, a provider can begin to form a partnership with the patient. But these partnerships must be balanced and authentic for a successful outcome. Providers need to ask the right questions. A good patient question to ask is, "What do you need right now?"

Key Ways a Provider Can Make a Difference

❧ Take extra time to ask where the patient is going on her disease journey. Explore with compassionate questions how the current illness began, how it has changed her life.

❧ Ask direct questions, such as, "How is this illness affecting you? How is it even protecting you? Is there a relationship either at home or at work that is not going well?" An illness can be a distraction from deeper life situations one is not able to confront or change.

❧ Invite your patient to reflect on the meaning of the disease and how she would like it to be different.

❧ Ask more questions about her needs— modalities such as water therapy, nutrition, energy work, homeopathic medicines, or counseling can help move her out of a stagnant state.

❧ Ask about relationships in the patient's life. Are they nourishing, significant relationships? Does she feel loved? Can she allow love in? Does she feel supported by friends, family, and loved ones?

❧ Ask what support around her would look like, what would it feel like to be supported.

Key Ways a Health Care Recipient (a Patient) Can Make a Difference

❧ See your practitioner as a medical partner who can help you explore what the disease brings to you, what you think and feel about the meaning of your disease.

❧ Share with your practitioner what you feel this illness represents to you, and how it makes you feel. Identify such feelings as anger, sadness, desperation, or grief, and speak about them.

❧ Rather than asking for medicines to suppress symptoms, ask for other forms of treatment that would help ease symptoms. Explore your intuition and be open to discovering the help needed for reduction or loss of symptoms.

❧ Consider what simple at-home remedies you could you do for yourself, such as soaking baths, increasing relaxation time, dancing, listening to music, art, meditating, or laughing more.

These ideas are not new; in fact, they are in use in some medical practices and by many women. To further improve the delivery of good, rational health care to people everywhere, we need to implement these ideas, and more like them, in the "doctor/patient relationship." Ask for this partnership approach – be straight forward. At the moment, we have a top-down approach that sends a message: the doctor (or entire medical system) knows what is best for you. Not always. A partnership can grow when communication improves; letting go of "just follow the doctor's orders" moves both sides forward.

The health care system is not the military; "following orders" is part of an archaic medical system that does not work for a twenty-first century population. It is far better to build consensus between the health-care recipient and the health-care practitioner. No one can know everything, but when we put our heads together, great ideas can emerge. The medical consulting room can provide a place to collaborate. Even in many urgent situations there is time to make level-headed consensus decisions. People need to be responsible for their lives and for the decisions they choose to make or not make.

The medical industry is a behemoth machine with tremendous power that strips away the patients' healing possibilities and rights the moment they step into a hospital or medical clinic. The way it has always been before no longer applies. Old ways of thinking and the old medical model must change and move into a more balanced, open minded, collaborative, insightful approach to health and well being.

Encouraging more input from the consumer, the patient; including other modalities; and using a team effort to find elegant solutions is essential for tapping into the inner healer.

Five Steps to Move Toward a Yin Paradigm:

1. Women recognize their significance and the value of their yin contributions.

As women recognize their value, the medical power balance will change. Stay-at-home moms often hang their heads when saying what they do, as if their work were unimportant. In my view, there is no work more important than raising children. Mothers are helping to shape a human being and building a responsible member of society. This is yin energy. Wiping noses, tending to skinned knees, and helping a child to learn about life is essential for the community to thrive. Women feed their families not only food, but also other nourishing ideas about life. They listen, they hold, they love. Tell me something that is more important than that. Women need to own this.

2. Women value their own voice.

Women's integrity and willingness to keep the family unit together give their voices value. For too long, women did not have the opportunity to speak in places of authority such as in government, courtrooms, and legislative bodies; for too long, women had no voting rights. Many women still do not hold equal professional status in academia, medicine, or law. Today a woman's voice is not equal to a man's. Some truths are emerging, yet many more need to follow. Woman's knowledge is valuable, practical, and life supporting. Women are finally shedding the old paradigms.

3. Place a greater focus on yin-based medicine.

Yin-based medicine would look very different. Patients would be in full charge of their health care. This would include planning or mapping a course of health maintenance, a way to keep health from declining. Numerous tools and supports are available to keep people healthy. In the allopathic (western/conventional) medical education system, physicians study primarily disease and pathology; very little, if any, medical education focuses on optimizing wellness, nutrition, and health. Just because these subjects are not taught in medical school does not make them less important. If you consult with a primary care doctor for disease care, balance that with a yin-focused provider, such as a well trained naturopathic physician, acupuncturist or chiropractor, to provide wellness care.

4. A team-based approach to wellness is the norm rather than an outlier.

When intelligent people form a team, magic can happen. Collaborative thinking and planning can yield spectacular ideas. Selecting and implementing various segments of the many healing modalities discussed can help patients move toward their goal. I experienced this concept in the early1980's when I worked with one of the first hospice teams in the U.S. The goal was to help the dying individual have the best possible quality of life right up until the end. The team included a physician, nurse, nurse's aide, spiritual counselor, social worker, and home volunteer. Each of us contributed to the wellbeing of our patients and their families.

We met weekly to review how the family was doing and what situations needed resolution. It was not perfect, but in the majority of cases, we each contributed to the whole. More important, the patient remained at home with family present when the transition to death occurred. No ego; we just wanted what was best for the patient. In my experience this was an outlier situation. Today we need to make this the norm for everyone. Teamwork works!

5. Change medical language to healing language.

"Fight" or "fighting" frequently appears in medical language relating to illness and recovery. Consider, for example, commonly heard phrases such as, "she's fighting for her life," or "she fought the battle to the end," or "you must fight this disease to survive." The idea of fighting is also a worldview concept and a common paradigm in western cultures, where it refers to staying ahead or to beating out another from seeking the top position. This idea of "fight" is part of the culture in the hierarchal system. In my view this idea of fighting disease does not belong in medicine.

Even with more integration of the softer modalities of medicine—chiropractic care, naturopathy, herbal remedies, homeopathy, and acupuncture—the dominant factor, the ego-centered direction, is still based in the model of fighting, conquering, winning...at all cost. The following military terms are found in western modern medical language; compare them to new words as they relate to illness.

Doctor's Orders	Restorative Plans or Doctor's Requests
Medical Officer	Health Provider
Fighting Disease	Making peace with illness
Barrage of treatments	Protective or supportive therapies
Invasion or invasive treatment	Infusion or soothing therapy
Natural killer cells	Savior cells
Conquer disease	Immune cell liberation
Attack	Coalesce healing
Defensive tactics or treatments	Collaborative treatments
War on cancer	Understanding cancer

Hierarchy vs. the Web

One person at the top who holds ultimate responsibility for all outcomes may work in such institutions as the military and church (where much of it began), but in medical care the model is failing its consumer. In emergency situations involving care protocols, a hierarchal structure has a benefit. But in the long-term care of individuals-the majority of medical situations-the hierarchy needs to change to a web-based paradigm.

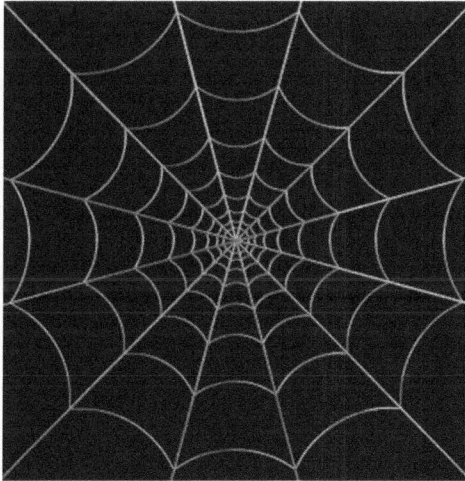

A web has a center, with radiating connections that are interrelated and interconnected. This is a perfect structure for care, and should be integrated into the entire health care system. A care team, with the patient at the center taking responsibility for care decisions, is the ideal. The person who is ill benefits from the collective thinking of the health care team. The support providers lend their expertise; most essential, there is communication of information among the entire team. In a case where patients cannot speak for themselves (coma, dementia, etc), the family, next of kin, or life partners have the advantage of the team's advice.

The Yin Yang Team

The ideal health-maintenance care team would include a clinician to provide and guide medical testing and physical exams, a nutritionist to provide specific dietary guidance, an exercise coach, and a life counselor or life coach. Optionally, the team might include a spiritual counselor or coach, a medical intuitive, and a body/energy worker. A team coordinator would take responsibility for directing the team to help fulfill the person's goals. Additionally, the medical record belongs to the patient, not to the medical organization. This approach would place responsibility where it belongs – with the individual. This team structure would lift the burden of full care and responsibility from the primary care provider by creating a partnership designed by and for the individual.

Health care has operated by under a set of controls that dictate who gets care, what the patient is told, the treatment choices, locally available treatment options, and treatment cost. By establishing equality and choices, selecting health team members with the patient, everything can change.

After years of being a witness, I have heard too many ultimatums given to patients in medical situations. The threat of dire consequences if a medical procedure is not done comes out of fear. The practitioner delivers it out of fear and the poor patient is often given only one maybe two choices of treatment. This is not a loving, nurturing, or positive situation. People have the right to decide what is best for them. Medical providers can and should only make the offer.

As the number of women in decision-making positions in the health profession continues to grow, this type of change is possible. Women contribute an essential aspect of life. Their yin qualities are needed. Let it begin in medicine by allowing recovery and balance to occur naturally. Let the yin voices rise and take an equal position with their yang counterparts. As the infusion of yin in medicine increases, it will permeate the community. People will feel more empowered in their health choices and their lives. "Alternative" modalities in the health movement will cease to be alternative; instead they will become part of the whole medical system.

21st Century Tale

Barbara

As a microbiology scientist, Barbara loves her work. But she began to feel concern when her eyesight became affected by the long-term medication she took. She was in danger of losing her sight and she needed other options. When she was 19, she learned she had rheumatoid arthritis, and she believed what she was told at the time: there was only one way to treat it. Even with ongoing drug therapy, she suffered unending joint pain and her physical limitations steadily increased. By the time she reached her 40's, she sometimes could not hold car keys with her right hand. That was disconcerting. What would the next 30 years be like, she wondered?

Her intuition suggested there had to be something else. A few years ago, she started learning about essential oils as gentle healers. Those she tried seemed to work for headaches and stress reduction. She asked whether there were other ways her body might heal. This last year, prompted by messages from her mind and heart, she began a course of more natural and safer healing modes.

After testing revealed that her intestinal tract had been damaged, she changed her entire nutritional program. That damage had led to the onset of her auto-immune disease. Now she follows the advice of and partners with a medically-trained naturopathic physician and is in significantly less pain. To her delight, she has increased joint mobility and is slowly recovering her strength and stamina

Looking back on her years of chronic pain and disability, she admits most times she knew her body better than the doctors, but was unable to trust any other process for managing her disease. Finally Barbara trusted her gut feeling to take charge of her own healing. She admits it has not been easy, but now knows she can trust her body to do its own healing. She is more empowered now than ever before. Her quality of life has significantly improved, and her next 30 (or more) years hold a greater promise.

✻

Wisdom of the Grandmothers: 21st Century Tale of Tales

The voices of women continue to rise; united feminine ideology and wisdom are stronger than ever before. Their voices join the chorus of wisdom keepers; the feminine, or yin, voice, strong , clear, and powerful. Grandmothers of the world are beginning to rise up and speak, including the **Thirteen Indigenous Grandmothers**, who have the wisdom to save the planet and have toured the world with their messages. They speak the yin of medicine—world medicine. Their message of peace and sustainable practices is for the next seven generations into the future.

A fitting end to this book is a portrait of hope. These Grandmothers are a group of women brimming with ancient wisdom who are teaching the importance of healing the planet. As women, they are deeply in touch with earth's wisdom. They have traveled from all over the world to speak to the world about healing. Through their global alliance, they are asking people to realize the impact each human has on the whole planet. Through prayer, education, as well as through healing thoughts, words, and actions, they send us their messages. Reverence for all creation is their theme. Through their worldwide work, people are opening to world healing. The grandmothers tell us that we must honor the indigenous cultural way, where every decision should be made with full awareness of its impact of the next seven generations and beyond. World healing starts with personal healing, and these revered women show us the way to our future. The grandmothers have respect for earth's sacred water and land, and compassion for all beings. See more about their work at http://www.grandmotherscouncil.org/.

Aama Bombo is a shaman, even though in her native Tamang people, in Nepal, women did not hold that role. After her father, also a shaman, passed, she received instructions from the spirits who guided her to follow his path. Grandmother Aama is currently well respected in her village; more than 100 people a day visit her to ask for help and healing. She prays, "I want to see this world full with natural beauty, where everybody will have equal rights and opportunity to share nature's womb."

Agnes Baker-Pilgrim is the eldest in her Takelma Indian tribe in southern Oregon. She says, "We can be the voice for the voiceless." Grandmother Agnes feels that if we create a vision in our hearts, it will spread. She believes, "As women of wisdom we cannot be divided."

Beatrice Long-Visitor Holy Dance is a great grandmother in her Lakota tribe. As a health worker she assists her people with diabetes. Grandmother Beatrice shares, "We use Indian Medicine all the time at home. Our spiritual ways, our Sun Dance ways, are encouraging prayer and bringing a lot of people back."

Bernadette Rebienot was born in Libreville in the Gabonese Republic of Africa. She is a leader in her community and a master of Women's Initiations. She has been the President of the Association of Traditional Practitioners of Gabonese Health since 1994. She says, "Nothing happens in my country without consulting the women."

Clara Shinolbu Iura, from Sao Paulo, Brazil, is a spiritual healer of prominence. Since 1999 she has directed the Santa Casa de Saude (Holy House of Health). Her belief is strong that through prayer, "...we may illuminate a consciousness for this planet."

Flordemayo was born in Central America and now resides in New Mexico. She gives lectures around the world as a part of the Wisdom of the Grandmothers Foundation. She believes we are at a crossroads and "... there is only one way to go to the light as a tribe."

Julieta Casimiro, a curandera and Mazatec elder from Oaxaca, Mexico, carries the tradition of healing and ceremonies. She says, "All of us here want the same thing. We want to walk in peace... and no more war."

Margaret Behan is President of the Cheyenne Elders Council and an accomplished writer, poet, and playwright. Grandmother Margaret says, "I know the ancient ways that we bring to this table from each of our traditions will make a difference."

Maria Alice Campos-Freire was born in Brazil and learned her sacred craft in the Amazon rainforest. After her spiritual teacher, Padrino Sebastiao, died, she began her journey around the world to share the teachings she learned.

She says, "Throughout time, prophecies have foretold that the moment of humanity's transmutation would arrive, and that women would be at the forefront of this process. And here we are, bringing our seed."

Mona Polacca is a Hopi/Havasupai/Tewa elder and now serves on several United Nations committees on indigenous people's issues. As CEO of the Turtle Island Project, she helps promote a wellness vision for her people. Grandmother Mona offers, "We Grandmothers, we have emerged from that darkness, see this beauty, see each other, and reach out to the world with open arms, with love, hope, compassion, faith, and charity. "

Rita Pitka Blumenstein was raised in Tununak, Alaska and schooled in Seattle, WA. She worked in health care many years, helping deliver babies. She leads "Talking Circles" healing conferences, and offers, "When we heal ourselves, we heal Mother Earth."

Rita Long-Visitor Holy Dance is a Lakota and a keeper of the traditional ways, which she teachers to children. She remembers going to Catholic boarding school and being forbidden to speak her native language. She tells us, "The planet needs to be taken care of; that includes all the people on this earth, not special groups."

Tsering Dolma Gyaltong, from Tibet, is a founding member of the Tibetan Women's Association. She helped establish over 30 branch offices worldwide and attended the Fourth Women's World Conference in Beijing, China. Grandmother Tsering tells us, "Our mind is what we have to be really happy within. If everyone really did a true spiritual practice, which develops into a positive mind, the world would not be in the dire situation we find it in today."

As we listen to the grandmothers' wisdom, we can begin to heal in multiple ways. We can feel our strength expand as we listen to their words and sense their deep, authentic caring. They are here to help us and to support the Great Mother. In this fast-paced world, the simple, the ordinary, and the sacred are often overlooked or forgotten. We must listen to the wise women of planet Earth. They are here to guide us and to show love and compassion for all beings.

Ancestors hold wisdom. The women who have traveled before us leave behind their lessons, as well as their gifts of strength, perseverance, and tenacity in the healing arts. They need us to continue the work they have begun. They leave us their voices.

My admiration of their work has grown beyond measure. Can we continue to carry the mantle of yin ways? I believe deep inside, women know the way. Now we can add our value and strength. We will be serving humanity.

～⊛～

Women once knew their place - and so do we.
Our home is the universe. Our task is anything we set
our minds and hearts to.
~ Maya V. Patel b. 1943

BIBLIOGRAPHY

Jeanne Achterberg, *Woman as Healer*, Boston, MA: Shambhala Publications, 1990.

Darlington, Cynthia, *The Female Brain*, Boca Raton, FL: CRC Press, 2009.

Charlotte Furth, *A Nourishing Yin*, Berkeley, CA: University of California Press, 1999.

Regina Markell Morantz-Sanchez, *Sympathy & Science*, New York: Oxford University Press, 1985.

Elizabeth Wright-Hubbard, MD, *Homeopathy as Art and Science*, Beaconsfield, Bucks UK: Beaconsfield Publishers LTD, 1990.

Elisabeth Brooke, *Women Healers*, Rochester, VT: Healing Arts Press, 1995.

Elisabeth Brooke, *Medicine Women: A Pictorial History of Women Healers*, Wheaton, IL: Quest Books, 1997.

Monica H. Green, *The Trotula*, Philadelphia: University of Pennsylvania Press, 2001.

Wighard Strehlow and Gottfried Hertzka, *Hildegard of Bingen's Medicine*, Santa Fe, NM: Bear & Co., 1988.

Barbara Montgomery Dossey, *Florence Nightingale, Mystic, Visionary, Healer*, Springhouse, Pennsylvannia: Springhouse Corporation, 2000.

Carol Shepherd McClain, *Women as Healers; Cross Cultural Perspectives*, New Brunswick, NJ: Rutgers University Press, 1995.

Jane B Donegon, *Hydropathic Highway to Health*, New York: Greenwood Press, 1986.

Jenny Sutcliffe and Nancy Duin, *A History of Medicine*, New York: Barnes & Noble, 1992.

Eliza Lo Chin, MD, *This Side of Doctoring: Reflections From Women In Medicine*, Thousand Oaks, CA: Sage Publications, 2002.

Laurie Scrivener and J. Suzanne Barnes, *A Biographical Dictionary of Women Healers, Midwives and Physicians*, Westport, CT: Oryx Press, 2002.

James Le Fanu MD, *The Rise and Fall of Modern Medicine*, New York: Carroll & Graf Publishers, 1999.

Elisabeth Kubler-Ross, *On Death and Dying*, New York: Touchstone, 1997.

Richard & Dorothy Wertz, *Lying-In: A History of Childbirth in America*, New York: Schocken Books, 1979.

Suzanne Arms, *Immaculate Deception II, Myth, Magic & Birth*, *Celestial Arts*, Berkeley, CA: Ten Speed Press, 1994.

Bobette Perrone, H. J. Henrietta Stockel and Victoria Krueger, *Medicine Women, Curanderas, and Women Doctors*, Oklahoma University Press, 1989.

Ted Kaptchuk, *The Web That Has No Weaver*, New York: Congdon & Weed, 1983.

Patricia Ebrey, *Chinese Civilization: A Sourcebook*, 2nd edition, New York: New York Free Press, 1993.

Martha Ostenso, *And They Shall Walk, The Life Story of Sister Elizabeth Kenny*, New York: Dodd Mead & Co., 1944.

Ellen S. Moore, *Restoring the Balance*, Cambridge, MA: Harvard University Press, 1999.

Kriste Lindenmeyer, *A Right to Childhood: the U.S. Children's Bureau and Child Welfare*, 1912-46, University of Illinois Press, 1997.

Ann K Boulis and Jerry Jacobs, *The Changing Face of Medicine*, Ithaca NY: Cornell University Press, 2008.

Mitchell Gaynor, MD, *Sounds of Healing*, New York: Broadway Books, 1999.

Louann Brizendine, MD, *The Female Brain*, New York: Broadway Books, 2006.

Danielle Ofri, MD, *Singular Intimacies: Becoming a Doctor at Bellevue, New York:* Penguin Books, 2004.

Mary Lefkowity and Maureen Fant, *Women's Life in Greece and Rome*, John Hopkins University Press, 1982.

Volney Steele, MD, *Bleed, Blister and Purge*, Missoula, MT: Mountain Press Publishing Co., 2005.

Merlin Stone, *When God Was A Woman*, New York: Harcourt, Inc, 1976.

Susan E. Cayleff, *Wash and Be Healed, The Water Cure Movement and Women's Health*, Philadelphia, PA: Temple University Press, 1987.

Carola Beresford-Cooke, *Shiatsu Theory and Practice*, New York: Churchill Livingstone, 1996.

Carl Dubitsky, *Bodywork Shiatsu*, Rochester, VT: Healing Arts Press, 1997.

Gaynor, Mitchell, *Healing Power of Sound*, Boston: Shambhala, 2002.

Barbara Tedlock, *The Woman in the Shaman's Body; Reclaiming the Feminine in Religion and Medicine*, New York: Bantam Books, 2005.

Kenneth Pelletier, *Mind as Healer, Mind as Slayer*, New York: Dell, 1977.

Douglas Bloch, *Words That Heal*, New York: Bantam Books, 1990.

Larry Dossey, *Healing Words*, San Francisco: Harper, 1993.

Ellen S. Moore, *Restoring the Balance: Women Physicians and Practice of Medicine* 1850-1995, Cambridge, MA: Harvard University Press, 2000.

Mary Chamberlain, *Old Wives' Tales; Their History, Remedies and Spells*, London: Virago Press, 1981.

Douglas Bloch, *Words That Heal*, Bantam Books, New York, 1990.

Shakti Gawain, *Living in the Light: A Guide to Personal and Planetary Transformation*, Novato, CA: New World Library, 1998.

ENDNOTES

[1] David Perlmutter, MD and Alberto Villoldo, PhD, *Power Up Your Brain: The Neuroscience of Enlightment,* Carlsbad, CA: Hay House, Inc., 2011, p. xxi.

[2] National College of Natural Medicine, Portland, OR, 14 Nov 2011, <www.ncnm.edu>.

[3] Alan Cohen, *A Deep Breath of Life*, Carlsbad, CA: Hay House, 1996.

[4] Early Healers, 14 Nov 2011, <http://www.btinternet.com/~ardena/early_healers.htm>.

[5] Ancient Egypt Online, *Gods of Ancient Egypt: Sekhmet,* 14 Nov 2011, <http://www.ancientegyptonline.co.uk/Sekhmet.html>.

[6] Theoi Greek Mythology: Exploring Mythology and the Greek Gods in Classical Literature and Art, *Agamede: Princess of Elis*, 14 Nov 2011, <http://www.theoi.com/Heroine/Agamede.html>.

[7] Jijith Nadumuri, Takshasila:The source of Ancient Knowledge, *Polydamma*, 20 Sep 2011, 14 Nov 2011, <http://takshasila.wikidot.com/ody:polydamna>.

[8] Jeanne Achterberg, *Woman as Healer,* Boston, MA: Shambhala Publications, 1990, p.32.

[9] Regina Markell Morantz-Sanchez, *Sympathy & Science,* New York: Oxford University Press, 1985, p. 28.

[10] Mary Chamberlain, *Old Wives Tales*, London: Virago Press, 1981, pp 36-42.

[11] Achterberg, op cit, p.30-31.

[12] Achterberg, op cit, p. 66.

[13] Adrienne Rich, *On Lies, Secrets and Silence: Selected prose 1966-1978*, New York: Norton, 1979.

[14] Chamberlain, *Old Wives Tales*, p. 4.

[15] Suzanne Arms, *Immaculate Deception II, Myth, Magic & Birth, Celestial Arts*, Berkeley, CA: Ten Speed Press, 1994, p.191.

[16] Index Mundi, *Infant Mortality Rate – Country Comparison*, 13 Mar 2012, <http://www.indexmundi.com/g/-r.aspx?c=xx&v=29>.

[17] Achterberg, op cit, pp 48-50.

[18] Elisabeth Brooke, *Women Healers*, Rochester, VT: Healing Arts Press, 1995, pp. 40-53.

[19] Wighard Strehlow and Gottfried Hertzka, *Hildegard of Bingen's Medicine*, Santa Fe, NM: Bear & Co., 1988, p. xxv-xxvi.

[20] Achterberg, op cit, p. 85.

[21] Yin – Yang, *The Meaning of Yin/Yang*, 16 Nov 2011, <http://fly.srk.fer.hr/~shlede/ying/yang.html>.

[22] Patricia Ebrey, *Chinese Civilization: A Sourcebook, 2d edition*, New York: Free Press, 1993, pp. 77-79.

[23] Charlotte Furth, *A Nourishing Yin*, Berkeley, CA: University of California Press, 1999, p 2.

[24] MedicineNet – Medicine and Health Information Produced by Doctors, *Definition of Allopathic medicine*, 22 Jan 2012, <http://www.medterms.com/script/main/art.asp?/articlekey=33612>.

[25] Furth, Charlotte, op. cit. p.13.

[26] Carol Shepherd McClain, *Women as Healers, Cross Cultural Perspectives*, New Brunswick, NJ: Rutgers University Press, 1995, pp 13, 25.

[27] McClain, op cit, p. 30.

[28] DONA International Research, *Birth Doulas Make a Difference*, 17 Nov 2011, <http://www.dona.org/resources/research.php#birth>.

[29] McClain, op cit, p. 42.

[30] The Social Welfare History Project, *Hamilton, Alic, M.D.*, 25 Jan 2012, <http://www.socialwelfarehistory.com/people/hamilton-alice-m-d/>.

[31] Barbara Montgomery Dossey, *Florence Nightingale, Mystic, Visionary, Healer*, Springhouse, Pennsylvannia: Springhouse Corporation, 2000, p. 186.

[32] New York Times: On This Day, *Miss Nightengale Dies, Aged Ninety*, 10 Mar 2012, <http://www.nytimes.com/learning/general/onthisday/bday/0512.html>.

[33] B. Dossey, op. cit. pp. 126-127.

[34] Ibid, p.199.

[35] Laurie Scrivener and J. Suzanne Barnes, *A Biographical Dictionary of Women Healers, Midwives and Physicians*, Westport, CT: Oryx Press, 2002, pp. 247-249.

[36] Dictionary.com, *Hierarchy*, 27 Feb 2012, <http://dictionary.reference.com/browse/hierarchy>.

[37] Advance for Nurses, *Nurses Want to Leave Hospitals Due to 'Moral Distress*,*'* 27 Feb 2012, <http://nursing.advanceweb.com/Article/Nurses-Want-to-Leave-Hospitals-Due-to-Moral-Distress.aspx>.

[38] Robert S. Mendelsohn MD, *Confessions of a Medical Heretic*, New York: Warner Books, 1979, p. 18-19.

[39] Anne Wilson-Schaef, *When Society Becomes An Addict*, San Francisco: Harper & Row, 1987, p.92.

[40]Jacques Jouanna, *Hippocrates*, Baltimore, MD: The John Hopkins University Press, 1999, p. 369.

[41] The Atlantic, *Medical Education in America*, 16 Nov 2012, <http://www.theatlantic.com/doc/191006/medical-education/2>.

[42] Elisabeth Brooke, *Medicine Women: A Pictorial History of Women Healers*, Wheaton, IL: Quest Books, 1997, p.59.

[43] B. Dossey, op cit, p. 320.

[44] Ibid, p. 321.

[45] Susan E. Cayleff, *Wash and Be Healed*, Philadelphia, PA: Temple University Press, 1987, p. 18.

[46] Ibid, p. 170.

[47] Ibid, p. 29.

[48] Volney Steele, MD, *Bleed, Blister and Purge*, Missoula, MT: Mountain Press Publishing Company, 2005, pp. 1-2.

[49] Cayleff, op.cit., p. 111.

[50] Ibid, p.110.

[51] Charles White MD, *Treatise on The Management of Pregnant and Lying In Women* (London 1773), reprint Science History Publications U.S.A., 1986.

[52] Jenny Sutcliffe and Nancy Duin, *A History of Medicine*, New York: Barnes & Noble, 1992, pp. 54-55.

[53] Ibid, p.55.

[54] Richard and Dorothy Wertz,, *Lying-In, a History of Childbirth in America*, New York: Schocken Books, 1979, p. 234.

[55] Andrew H. Beck, *The Flexner Report and the Standardization of American Medical Education*, JAMA, 2004; 291:2139-2140.

[56] Ibid, p. 2139.

[57] Achterberg, op. cit. p. 147.

[58] Achterberg, op.cit. p 154.

[59] Regina Markell Morantz, *Feminism, Professionalism, and Germs: The Thought of Mary Putnam Jacobi and Elizabeth Blackwell*, American Quarterly, Vol. 34, No 5 (Winter 1982), pp. 459-478.

[60] Mary Putnam Jacobi, *Shall Women Practice Medicine*, The North American Review, Vol. 134, No. 302 (Jan., 1882), pp. 52-75.

[61] Boyle and Friedhelm, *Nature Doctors*, East Palestine, OH: Buckeye Naturopathic Press, 1994, p. 221.

[62] Ibid, pp. 221-224.

[63] Ibid, p. 225.

[64] Sutcliffe and Duin, op.cit. p. 81.

[65] Regina Markell Morantz-Sanchez, *Sympathy & Science*, New York: Oxford University Press, 1985, p. 64.

[66] Merlin Stone, *When God Was A Woman*, New York: Harcourt, Inc, 1976, p. 3.

[67] Achterberg, op cit, p. 14.

[68] Ibid, p. 28.

[69] Louann Brizendine, MD, *The Female Brain,* New York: Broadway Books, 2006, p. 102.

[70] Achterberg, op cit, p. 107.

[71] Vaccination Liberation – Information, *Smallpox Inoculation - A Timeline with Comments*, 25 Jan 2012, <http://www.vaclib.org/basic/smallpox.htm>.

[72] Donald R. Hopkins, *Princes and Peasants: Smallpox in History*, University of Chicago Press, 1983, page not found.

[73] Achterberg, op.cit., p. 109.

[74] The Changing Face of Medicine, *Dr. Bernadine Healy*, 13 Mar 2012, <http://www.nlm.nih.gov/changingthefaceofmedicine/physicians/biography_145.html>.

75 Ibid.

76 Early Childhood Education Journal, *Beneficial Effects of Tactile Stimulation*, Volume 27, Number 4, pp. 255-257.

77 Dolores Krieger, *The Therapeutic Touch: How to Use Your Hands to Help or to Heal,* Englewood Cliffs, NJ: Prentice-Hall, Inc, 1979, p. vii-viii.

78 Susan Wager, MD, *Doctor's Guide to Therapeutic Touch,* New York: Berkley Publishing Group, 1996, p. viii.

79 Krieger, op. cit., pp. 18-19.

80 Jeffery Fisher, Marvin Rytting and Richard Heslin, *Hands Touching Hands, Affective and Evaluative Effects of an Interpersonal Touch,* Sociometry, Vol. 39, No. 4, pp. 416-421.

81 Carola Beresford-Cooke, *Shiatsu Theory and Practice*, New York: Churchill Livingstone, 1996, p.1.

82 Carl Dubitsky, *Bodywork Shiatsu*, Rochester, VT: Healing Arts Press, 1997, p. 4.

83 Hands to Heart International, 14 Nov 2011, <http://www.handstohearts.org>.

84 Barbara Tedlock, *The Woman in the Shaman's Body; Reclaiming the Feminine in Religion and Medicine,* New York: Bantam Dell, 2005, p.15

85 Tedlock, ibid, p.16

86 Mitchell Gaynor, MD, *Sounds of Healing,* New York: Broadway Books, 1999, p. 36.

87 Ibid, p. 82.

88 Ibid, p. 38.

89 Douglas Bloch, *Words That Heal,* New York: Bantam Books, 1990, p. 19.

90 Kenneth Pelletier, *Mind as Healer, Mind as Slayer,* New York: Dell, 1977, pp. 191-192.

[91] Larry Dossey, *Healing Words: The Power of Prayer and the Practice of Medicine*, San Francisco: Harper San Francisco, 1993, p. 10.

[92] *American Heritage Dictionary of the English Language*, Fourth Edition, Houghton Mifflin Company, 2009.

[93] Centers for Disease Control and Prevention, *National Center for Health Statistics*, 18 Oct 2011, <http://www.cdc.gov-/nchs/>, retrieved October 18, 2011.

[94] *Stedman's Medical Dictionary, 27th edition*, Lippincott, Williams and Wilkins, 2000.

[95] Biomed Central: BMC Pallative Care, *Factors associated with home death for individuals who receive home support services: a retrospective cohort study*, 14 Nov 2011, <http://www.biomed-central.com/1472-684X/1/2/>.

[96] Mary E. Lauer, Raymond K. Mulhern, Joyce M. Wallskog, and Bruce M. Camitta, Pediatrics, *A Comparison Study of Parental Adaptation Following a Child's Death at Home or in the Hospital*, 14 Nov 2011, <http://pediatrics.aappublications.org/cgi/content/abstract/71/1/107>.

[97] Siamak Nabili, MD, MPH, MedicineNet.com, *What is a Hospitalist*, 14 Nov 2011, <http://www.medicinenet.com/-script/main/art.asp?articlekey=93946>.

[98] Medscape, *Another In-Hospital CV Risk Marker: 24-Hour Shifts with Overnight On-Call Duty*, 17 Nov 2011, <http://www.medscape.com/viewarticle/711835>.

[99] Gary Null PhD, Carolyn Dean MD ND, Martin Feldman MD, Debora Rasio MD and Dorothy Smith PhD,   A Theory of Civilization, *The American Medical System is the Leading Cause of Death and Injury in the United States*, 14 Nov 2011, <http://www.ourcivilisation.com/medicine/ usamed.htm>.

[100] Quick, Jonathan, Critical Information in a Flash!, *The American Medical System is the Leading Cause of Death in the US-*

Part 3 of 6: Medical Ethics and Conflict of Interest in Scientific Medicine, 11 Apr 2011, 22 Nov 2011, <http://curatiokey.com/-blog/the-american-medical-system-is-the-leading-cause-of-death-in-the-us-part-3-of-6/>.

[101] Elisabeth Brooke, *Women Healers: Portraits of Herbalists, Physicians, and Midwives,* Rochester, VT: Healing Arts Press, 1995, p. 99.

[102] Ibid, pp. 101-103.

[103] Changing the Face of Medicine, *Dr. Lillie Rosa Minoka-Hill,* 12 Mar 2012, <http://www.nlm.nih.gov/changingthe face-ofmedicine/physicians/biography_226.html>.

[104] Society for Participatory Medicine, 29 Feb 2012, <http://participatorymedicine.org>.

[105] Darlington, Cynthia, *The Female Brain,* Boca Raton, FL: CRC Press, 2009, p. 234.

[106] Darlington, op cit, pp. 91- 92.

[107] A hormone dominant in females that intensifies uterine contractions, stimulates milk "let-down", and allows women to bond with their children.

[108] Louann Brizendine, MD, *The Female Brain,* New York: Broadway Books, 2006, p. 41.

[109] Ibid, p.42.

[110] Brizendine, op cit, pp 67-68.

[111] Shelley E. Taylor, Laura Cousino Klein, Brian P Lewis, Tara L, Gruenewald, Regan A. R. Gurung, John A. Updegraff, *Biobehavioral Responses to Stress in Females: Tend-and-Befriend, Not Fight-or-Flight,* Psychological Review, Vol. 107(3), Jul 2000, pp. 411-429.

[112] Grief.com: Because Love Never Dies, *Elisabeth Kübler-Ross,* 27 Jan 2012, <http://grief.com/elisabeth-kubler-ross/>.

[113] It's In Our Touch: Hospice of Montgomery, *Cicely Saunders and the Modern Hospice Movement*, 16 Dec 08, 27 Jan 2012, <http://www.hospiceofmontgomery.org /en/art/6/>.

[114] Ibid.

[115] Danielle Ofri, *Singular Intimacies: Becoming a Doctor at Bellevue*, New York: Penguin Books, p. 234.

[116] Rinpoche Sogyal, *The Tibetan Book of Living and Dying*, San Francisco: Harper, 1992.

[117] Random House Dictionary, 2nd edition, New York: Random House, 1987.

[118] Eliza Lo Chin, MD, *This Side of Doctoring: Reflections From Women In Medicine*, Thousand Oaks, CA: Sage Publications, 2002, p. 8.

[119] Title IX states: "No person in the U.S. shall, on the basis of sex, be excluded from participation in, or denied the benefits of, or be subjected to discrimination under any educational program or activity receiving federal aid."

[120] Pauline W. Chen, MD, *Do Women Make Better Doctors?*, New York Times, May 6, 2010.

[121] Debra L, Roter, PhD, Judith A, Hall, PhD and Yutaka Aoki, MS, MHS, ME, *Physician Gender Effects in Medical Communication—A Meta-Analytic Review*, JAMA 2002: 288(6) 756-764.doi.

[122] Bosworth and Schaie, *The Relationship of Social Environment, Social Networks, and Health Outcomes*, Journal of Gerontology: Psychological Sciences, 1997, Vol. 52B, No. 5, pp. 197-205.

[123] L. Frank Schnell, *The Philosophy and Principles of Naturopathic Medicine*, original manuscript, Calgary, Canada, 1968, p. 47.

[124] Henry Beecher, MD, *The Powerful Placebo*, JAMA 1955; 15a(17):1602-1606.doi

[125] Michael Pollan, New York Times, *Unhappy Meals*, 28 Jan 2007, 14 Nov 2011, <www.nytimes.com/2007/01/-28/magazine/28nutritionism.t.html>.

[126] Jonas Mosby, *Jonas Mosby's Dictionary of Complementary and Alternative Medicine*, Elsevier, 2005.

[127] The Institute for Functional Medicine, 27 Jan 2012, <http://www.functionalmedicine.org/>.

[128] Barbara Ehrenreich and Deidre English, *For Her Own Good: 150 Years of the Experts' Advice to Women*, New York: Anchor/Doubleday and Co, 1978, p. 292.

[129] Gabor Maté, 16 Nov 2011, <http://drgabormate.com>.

[130] Random House Dictionary of the English Language 2nd edition – Unabridged,

New York: Random House, 1987.

[131] Journal of Psychosomatic Research, 29 Jan 2012, <http://www.jpsychores.com/article/S0022-3999(99)00091-4/abstract>.

www.ingramcontent.com/pod-product-compliance
Lightning Source LLC
Chambersburg PA
CBHW031512270326
41930CB00006B/372